Evidence Based Dentistry for Effective Practice

Edited by

Jan Clarkson BDS, BSc, PhD, FDS (Paed), RCSEd
Dental Health Services Research Unit
Dundee Dental Hospital and School
University of Dundee
Dundee, UK

Jayne E Harrison BDS, FDS (Orth), RCPS, MOrth RCS Ed,
MDentSci, PhD
Department of Clinical Dental Sciences
Liverpool University Dental Hospital
Liverpool, UK

Amid I Ismail BDS, MPH, DrPH
Department of Cariology
Restorative Sciences and Endodontics
School of Dentistry
University of Michigan
Ann Arbor, Michigan, USA

Ian Needleman BDS, MSc, PhD, MRD, RCS, RCPS, DGDP (UK)
Department of Periodontology
Eastman Dental Institute for Oral Health Care Sciences
University College London
London, UK

Helen Worthington PhD, MSc, CStat
Cochrane Oral Health Group
University Dental Hospital of Manchester
Manchester, UK

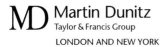

Martin Dunitz
Taylor & Francis Group

LONDON AND NEW YORK

© 2003 Martin Dunitz, an imprint of the Taylor & Francis Group

First published in the United Kingdom in 2003
by Martin Dunitz, an imprint of the Taylor & Francis Group, 11 New Fetter Lane,
London EC4P 4EE

Tel.: +44 (0) 20 7583 9855
Fax.: +44 (0) 20 7842 2298
E-mail: info@dunitz.co.uk
Website: http://www.dunitz.co.uk

Although every effort has been made to ensure that all owners of copyright material have been acknowledged in this publication, we would be glad to acknowledge in subsequent reprints or editions any omissions brought to our attention.

The views expressed in this book are those of the individual authors and do not necessarily represent those of the institutions where the contributing authors are employed.

A CIP record for this book is available from the British Library.

ISBN 1 84184 199 4

Distributed in the USA by:
Thieme Medical Publishers Inc
333 Seventh Avenue
New York, NY 10001
USA
Tel: +1 212 760 0888

Distributed in the rest of the world by:
Thomson Publishing Services
Cheriton House
North Way
Andover, Hampshire SP10 5BE, UK
Tel.: +44 (0)1264 332424
E-mail: salesorder.tandf@thomsonpublishingservices.co.uk

Composition by Wearset Ltd, Boldon, Tyne and Wear

Printed and bound in Great Britain by The Cromwell Press, Trowbridge

Contents

Contributors

Sylvia R Bickley
Cochrane Oral Health Group
University Dental Hospital of
Manchester
Higher Cambridge Street
Manchester M15 6FH, UK

Brian C Bonner
Dental Health Services Research
Unit
Dundee Dental Hospital and
School
University of Dundee
Park Place
Dundee DD1 4HR, UK

Jan Clarkson
Dental Health Services Research
Unit
Dundee Dental Hospital and
School
University of Dundee
Park Place
Dundee DD1 4HR, UK

Iain K Crombie
Department of Epidemiology and
Public Health
Ninewells Hospital and Medical
School
Dundee DD1 9SY, UK

Julian PL Davis
Department of Epidemiology and
Public Health
Ninewells Hospital and Medical
School
Dundee DD1 9SY, UK

Chris Deery
Edinburgh Dental Institute
Children's Department
Lauriston Building
3 Lauriston Place
Edinburgh EH3 9YW, UK

Anne-Marie Glenny
Cochrane Oral Health Group
Manchester Dental Education
Centre
University Dental Hospital of
Manchester
Higher Cambridge Street
Manchester M15 6FH, UK

Jeremy Grimshaw
Clinical Epidemiology
Programme
Centre for Best Practice
Institute of Population Health
Ottawa Health Research Institute
1053 Carling Avenue
Ottawa, Ontario K1Y 4E9, Canada

Jayne E Harrison
Department of Clinical Dental
Sciences
Liverpool University Dental
Hospital and School of Dentistry
Pembroke Place
Liverpool L3 5PS, UK

Lee Hooper
Cochrane Oral Health Group
Manchester Dental Education
Centre
University Dental Hospital of
Manchester
Higher Cambridge Street
Manchester M15 6FH, UK

Bob Ireland
Department of Clinical Dental
Sciences
Liverpool University Dental
Hospital and School of Dentistry
Pembroke Place
Liverpool L3 5PS, UK

Amid Ismail
Department of Cariology
Restorative Sciences and
Endodontics D 2347
University of Michigan School of
Dentistry
Ann Arbor MI 48109–1078, USA

Sabina Kasem
Department of Orthodontics
University Dental Hospital
Manchester
Higher Cambridge Street
Manchester M15 6FM

Hiroshi Miyashita
EndoPerio Specialist Dental Clinic
Aoyama-Marutake bdg 4F
3-1-36 Minami-Aoyama
Minato-Ku
Tokyo 107-0062, Japan

Ian Needleman
Department of Periodontology
Eastman Dental Institute for Oral
Health Care Sciences
University College London
256 Gray's Inn Road
London WC1X 8LD, UK

Nigel Pitts
Dental Health Services Research
Unit
Dundee Dental Hospital and
School
University of Dundee
Park Place
Dundee DD1 4HR, UK

Jim Rennie
NHS Education for Scotland
Hanover Buildings
66 Rose Street
Edinburgh EH2 2NN, UK

Anwar Ali Shah
Unit of Orthodontics
Division of Oral Health and
Development School of Clinical
Dentistry
University of Sheffield
Sheffield S10 2TA, UK

Bill Shaw
Manchester Dental Education
Centre
University Dental Hospital of
Manchester
Higher Cambridge Street
Manchester M15 6FH, UK

Emma Tavender
Cochrane Oral Health Group
Manchester Dental Education
Centre
University Dental Hospital of
Manchester
Higher Cambridge Street
Manchester M15 6FH, UK

Helen Worthington
Cochrane Oral Health Group
University Dental Hospital of
Manchester
Manchester Science Park
Lloyd Street North
Manchester M15 4SH, UK

Acknowledgement

The editors would like to express their sincere appreciation and thanks to Diane Lynas for facilitating the production of this book.

Foreword

Dentistry has many drivers and the last few decades have seen one aspect of science, namely material science and technology, driving practice in remarkable ways. In the last decade, however, another aspect of science has started to drive change, an approach called 'evidence based decision-making'.

The first scientific revolution assumed that better technology led to better outcome and was relatively uncritical about methods used to assess the improvement of outcome. However, the second scientific revolution, sometimes called the 'evidence based decision-making revolution', started to raise issues not only about the amount of evidence that was available but also its quality. New technological developments are often startling, and it may appear to be churlish to question the evidence on which they are based, but the concept that evidence has a quality as well as a quantity has changed the face of decision-making. Much more attention is being paid to the quality of evidence on which decisions are based, either at national policy-making level or in relation to individual patients.

Evidence is global but its application is local, be that national, within a practice, or for an individual patient, and evidence based clinical practice is that in which decisions are applied to help individual patients. Evidence based healthcare and public health, in which the evidence is applied to populations, require a set of skills that has not been conventionally included in professional training.

This book sets out the new agenda and describes the new scientific revolution concerned with the quality as well as the quantity of evidence.

A third revolution is now apparent and that is the revolution that will be led by patients. At present patients are too often inarticulate and uninformed, particularly in dentistry, where the proportion of time taken to discuss decisions with patients is probably less than in any other clinical specialty. Based on work done in screening, the resourceful patient of the 21st century has been described as one who, using the Internet, will be of importance to dentistry in two ways: individual dentists will have to take the patient's preferred style of decision-making into account when discussing options for expensive treatment; and patients may prove to be the mainspring of change. The advocates of evidence based decision-making, who often face apathy or even hostility from other clinical colleagues, may find the resourceful patient of the 21st century their main ally.[1]

JA Muir Gray, CBE, DSc, MD, FRCP, FRCPSGlas
Oxford

1. Muir Gray JA, *The Resourceful Patient* (Rosetta Press: Park Ridge, 2002).

chapter 1

Introduction to evidence based dentistry

Ian Needleman

Introduction

> But what is so special about medicine? We are, through the media, as
> ordinary citizens, confronted daily with controversy and debate
> across a whole spectrum of public policy issues. But typically, we have
> no access to any form of systematic 'evidence base' – and therefore no
> means of participating in the debate in a mature and informed
> manner. Obvious topical examples include education – what does
> work in the classroom? – and penal policy – what is effective in pre-
> venting re-offending?[1]

Dentists striving to offer the best quality of care for their patients take
decisions on diagnosis, prognosis and clinical management based on
evidence. The evidence may be good, up to date and appropriate for the
patient or it may not be. Knowing whether the evidence is valid and
usable is fraught with uncertainty. Further pressures on good evidence
use are the rapid increase in the amount of published research, the
emphasis on quality assurance and clinical governance and the introduction of mandatory continuing professional education in many countries.

Helping the clinician to maximize the use of 'best' available evidence
is what evidence based practice (EBP) is all about. EBP helps to translate
a particular clinical problem into a question that can be answered

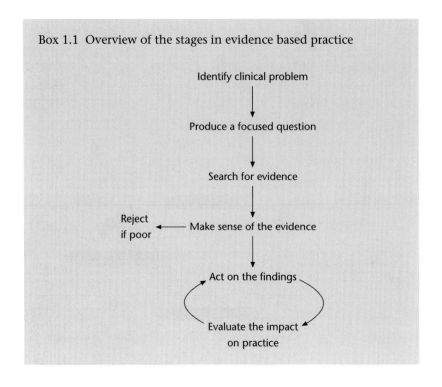

Box 1.1 Overview of the stages in evidence based practice

Identify clinical problem

↓

Produce a focused question

↓

Search for evidence

↓

Reject if poor ←——— Make sense of the evidence

↓

Act on the findings

Evaluate the impact on practice

(Box 1.1). The answer takes the form of a systematic approach to tracking down relevant information, followed by an appraisal of the quality and validity of the research. As a result, the core of decision making in medicine and dentistry is aided by a systematic appreciation of the relevant data. In this chapter I will present an overview of evidence based practice as it relates to dentistry and look in more detail at the first skill of EBP, that is, the asking of clinically relevant questions. Following this, I will present a brief history of EBP and the development of EBP activity in dentistry. For the purpose of this chapter, and for simplicity, I will use the term evidence based practice to cover evidence based health care as it relates to clinical patient management in dentistry and medicine.

EBP as decision support

The definition that encapsulates EBP best is 'An approach to decision making in which the clinician uses the best evidence available, in consultation with the patient, to decide upon the option which suits that patient best'[2] (Box 1.2).

Evidence based practice is therefore a means of decision support in clinical practice, and not simply a formula to drive clinical management without consideration of the patient. In other words, highly developed clinical skills and experience are essential to the correct use of EBP.

Box 1.2 Relationship of clinical skills, the patient and the 'evidence' to evidence based dentistry

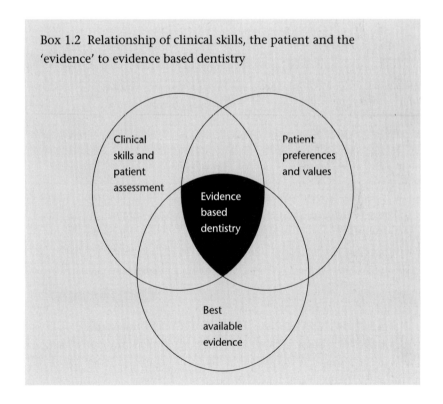

Evidence based practice or practice based on evidence?

Most clinicians will correctly feel that their practice is already built upon evidence, and some may be concerned that EBP is therefore an attack on their professionalism. I will call traditional dental practice 'based on evidence practice'. It makes substantial use of evidence, but the use of evidence is selective and may therefore be biased, incomplete, out of date or all three. Instead, EBP provides clinicians with a systematic evidence base and a greater security in reaching healthcare decisions.

EBP vs traditional practice

To help understand EBP further, I will compare EBP with a traditional model of dental practice as illustrated in Box 1.3. Both approaches have in common the need for well-developed clinical skills and clinical

---

Box 1.3 Comparison of EBP vs traditional practice

Evidence based practice	*Traditional practice*
Similarities	
• High value of clinical skills and experience	
• Fundamental importance of integrating evidence with patient values	
Differences	
• Uses best evidence available	• Unclear basis of evidence
• Systematic appraisal of quality of evidence	• Unclear or absent appraisal of quality of evidence
• More objective, more transparent and less biased process	• More subjective, more opaque and more biased process
• Greater acceptance of levels of uncertainty	• Greater tendency to black and white conclusions

experience. These skills include accurate history taking, methodical examination procedures and rational approaches to diagnosis.

EBP and traditional approaches differ in their use of evidence. EBP attempts to locate and use the best available evidence through a search that has been systematic and thorough. This systematic approach should minimize the potential bias of selecting only data that support a particular viewpoint. In addition, once the research has been identified, the quality and applicability to particular patient types is assessed. Since both good and bad research exist in print, critical appraisal is essential. Furthermore, by ensuring that the methods by which an evidence based conclusion has been reached are transparent, each reader can be in the position of evaluating the validity of the conclusions. EBP should therefore give dentists greater confidence in the basis of clinical decisions.

Uncertainty in decision making

One trade-off for evidence based practice is that uncertainty is more explicitly acknowledged. An example of this is the use of the term 'best' evidence. Best does not always mean a high level of evidence, but simply what is the best available for a particular question or problem. Research designs vary in their strength of evidence. Put another way, the ability to demonstrate that, for instance, one treatment is better than another or that one factor is the causative agent for a disease over another factor, varies with study design and will be addressed more fully in Chapter 2. EBP evaluates the type and quality of the research and indicates to the reader the strength of the evidence. I have illustrated this with some examples from the recently published Scottish Intercollegiate Guidelines Network (SIGN) guideline on management of unerupted and impacted third molar teeth (Box 1.4).[3]

A further example of uncertainty is that an evidence based conclusion may take the form of a probability rather than a black and white conclusion as to whether a treatment works or not. Indeed, no treatment is 100% predictable in its outcome. For example, we recently conducted a systematic review of the effectiveness of a relatively new periodontal

---

Box 1.4. Selections from SIGN guideline of third molar extraction

I have selected three sample recommendations to illustrate the range of grades of recommendations from A–C. Clearly, the evidence is strong for the use of postoperative steroids and weak for autologous transplantation of third molars.[3]

Grade/Clinical recommendations
    Removal of unerupted and impacted third molars is *not* advisable:
B   In patients with deeply impacted third molars and no history of evidence of pertinent local or systemic pathology

    Other indications for third molar removal:
C   For autologous transplantation to a first molar socket

    Clinical management (following extraction):
A   Preoperative steroid should be considered (unless contraindicated) where there is a risk of significant postoperative swelling

Grades of recommendation
A   Requires at least one randomized controlled trial as part of a body of literature of overall good quality and consistency addressing the specific recommendation.
B   Requires the availability of well-conducted clinical studies but no randomized clinical trials on the topic of recommendation.
C   Requires evidence obtained from expert committees reports or opinions and/or clinical experiences of respected authorities. Indicates an absence of directly applicable clinical studies of good quality.

---

surgical procedure called guided tissue regeneration compared to the current standard form of surgery (control treatment).[4] On the whole the results demonstrated a 1.1 mm greater gain in attachment for the new treatment compared with conventional surgery. However, this statistic was not very informative about the predictability of achieving the benefit. Therefore we also calculated the number of sites that would need to be treated (NNT) with guided tissue regeneration in order to obtain one site with a meaningful significant clinically superior result over control therapy. The results indicated that eight sites would need to be treated in this manner, indicating quite a high level of uncertainty of beneficial effect. Therefore we have taken a relatively uninformative overall estimate of clinical effect (the mean value) and translated this into an estimate of the certainty of actually achieving a benefit.

Whilst this might appear at first sight to hinder the decision making process, it should help by being more informative about the likely chances of benefits (about which many patients ask); it can also be examined in different patients to highlight when a treatment is most likely to help. Finally, acknowledging and interpreting the uncertainty that always exists in dentistry is a more honest use of research data.

Turning clinical problems into answerable questions – the first step in evidence based practice

The first skill in EBP is designing a well-built clinical question.[5] These are some scenarios from the life of a busy dentist:

At a trade show, you are considering buying an apex locator to aid your endodontic diagnosis. You are unsure how accurate these devices are and whether to believe the trade representative's comments.

The following day, you are treating a 50-year-old woman with periodontal disease who smokes 20 cigarettes per day. You wonder whether you should boost the effect of the root planing with locally applied antibiotics.

Later in the day you receive the biopsy report of a 39-year-old man confirming your clinical diagnosis of lichen planus. You consider what information you should give him about the risk of malignancy from the condition.

Finally, in the evening, it is your turn to chair your local peer-review group. Your colleagues have kindly nominated you to give a short presentation on effective methods for preventing root caries.

These questions illustrate real dilemmas in diagnosis, therapy, prognosis and prevention. To find reliable answers efficiently is the skill of a focused questioner. The advantage of setting a focused question is that it helps to clarify in your mind what you really want or need to answer. As a result it becomes easier to determine the type of evidence that is needed for the answer and thus to search for it efficiently. I will illustrate this below.[6] Without a focused question, you may not be entirely sure exactly what you are asking and your question may in fact be a series of questions or not really answerable. To help develop the focused question, a framework exists that will help you to define the problem. The framework breaks the question into four components, Patient, Intervention, Comparison and Outcomes, and is known by the acronym PICO (Box 1.5). Breaking the question into its component parts makes it much easier to focus on the aspects of answering the problem that really interest you. A further advantage is that it makes it easier for you or your friendly librarian (information manager) to design an efficient search, as you will see in Chapter 2.

Let me illustrate this with a real example that cropped up in my practice. As a periodontist, I spend increasing amounts of time providing smoking cessation advice to my patients. Towards the end of 2000, a new smoking cessation therapy was licensed in the UK called bupropion (Zyban). It is taken systemically and has a different mode of action from nicotine replacement therapy, which I already knew from previous searching was an effective, evidence based therapy.[7] In addition, the claims for bupropion were impressive and clearly I needed to find out

Box 1.5 Format of a structured question using the PICO layout

Patient/problem	Intervention	Comparison	Outcome
What is a concise description of the particular patient or problem?	Which main treatment am I considering?	Am I comparing the treatment against the best alternative or no treatment?	What is (are) the main outcome(s) that interests my patient and me?

whether I should incorporate this into my practice. The basic question was 'Does bupropion work?' but what did this really mean?

Identifying the problem or patient was straightforward. I was interested in smokers and in particular heavier smokers with greater nicotine dependence. The intervention was also straightforward as I was looking specifically at bupropion. For the comparison I was interested in nicotine replacement therapy since this was the best option at the time. For outcomes, I was interested not only in the positive measures (quit rate) but also in any significant side effects (Box 1.6). After re-assembling the PICO into a coherent question, it becomes 'In moderate to heavy smokers, what is the effect of bupropion compared with nicotine replacement therapy in quit rates at 12 months, and what are the main adverse effects?'

My first step (as always) was to see if there were any good systematic reviews since the data would be quality appraised. I looked at the Cochrane Library and found two reviews that gave me the answers.[7,8] These reviews told me that only one clinical trial has compared bupropion with nicotine patches. The results showed a significant advantage for the new therapy for quit rates at 12 months (odds ratio 2.07, 95% CI: 1.22, 3.53). Adverse effects included a risk of seizures of 1/1000 (which is the same rate as any antidepressant) and insomnia in 30–40% of patients. I was also interested to see the occurrence of dry mouth in 10% of the patients as this could impact on periodontal therapy. The conclusions of the review were that, while bupropion is recommended as a first line treatment, there was currently insufficient published evidence to recommend it over nicotine replacement therapy, but that bupropion might be helpful in those who fail to quit as a result of nicotine replacement therapy.

Box 1.6 Bupropion question in a PICO format

Problem/patient	Intervention	Comparison	Outcome
Moderate/heavy smokers (>10 day)	Bupropion	Nicotine replacement therapy	1. Quit rates 2. Adverse effects

The process from question to answer took me about 45 minutes, which was within my usual remit of 'Can I do this during a lunchtime?' For those without ready access to the Cochrane Library, I also found the information within a further 10 minutes through a search engine using the term 'Zyban'. This was located within the US Surgeon General's latest clinical practice guideline.[9] If I had not found the systematic review or evidence based guideline, I could have conducted a MEDLINE search and looked at original clinical trial reports or examined traditional, non-systematic reviews. At that stage, involving a librarian in the search might have been sensible in order to help locate the information.

Problems with focused questions

Two problems frequently crop up when starting to develop these skills. The first problem occurs when a question is so specific that there is no available answer for that exact, narrow question. If this is the case, examine each component (usually the patient or problem) to see if it is reasonable to accept a broader definition. Or put another way, is there a good reason to think that a broader group of patients would respond differently from the individual patient who precipitated this question? Another problem that can occur with a patient with multiple problems is knowing where to start. This is really no different from conventional treatment planning and you should use your clinical skills to prioritize these. This may be on the basis of clinical urgency or careful listening to the patient to understand why they have really come to see you. Designing and answering focused questions can be an excellent foundation to the activities of a study club or peer-review group.

Development of EBP

Many strands in medicine and dentistry have contributed to what is now termed EBP and it is probably not sensible to try to trace a direct lineage. Swales explores the development of three medical cultures and their virulent reaction to one another.[10] Each was also passionate about the correctness of their approach. The three schools were: clinical methods (practice by experience and anecdote), pathophysiology (laboratory based experimental science) and the numerical method which later developed into clinical epidemiology and then into EBP. In 19th century France, Claude Bernard preached that pathophysiological processes were paramount. He concluded that there was little place in medical progress for clinical observations on individuals or populations. Protagonists of clinical methods or the art of medicine were not always convinced. Their reaction to adopting the German model of academic clinicians in London Medical schools was quoted as 'treating hospital patients as a form of experimental reagent'.[10]

The numerical method was championed by Pierre Louis (b. 1787). During his service as Physician to the Czar, Louis became disillusioned with medicine when he observed a lack of understanding of the treatment and prevention of cholera. He returned to Paris for further study but concluded that the level of knowledge and education of his teachers was unsatisfactory and rather than learning from didactic lessons, he took the then novel step of making careful observations of the effect of treatment on patients. He collected the data together and tabulated the information. Louis stated that 'a therapeutic agent cannot be employed with any discrimination or probability of success in a given case, unless its general efficacy, in analogous cases, has been previously ascertained'.[11]

His most celebrated work challenged the routine practice of bleeding to treat inflammatory conditions such as typhoid. Bleeding was considered a first line treatment since the pathophysiologists had noted that inflammation was associated with increased blood flow (which was a correct observation) but concluded that bleeding was therefore therapeutic (which was an incorrect assumption). The numerical method generated much hostility. Practising physicians were unwilling to discard therapies 'validated by both tradition and their own experience on account of somebody else's numbers'.[12] In addition, the use of aggregated facts, rather than interest in the individual, was perceived as questioning the humanitarianism of the medical profession.

It would be wrong to give the impression that these arguments are historical only. In recent decades, some treatments based on clinical traditional and pathophysiological sense alone have subsequently been shown to be ineffective once subject to a clinical trial. For example, for many years anti-arrhythmic drugs were used to control ventricular extrasystole following myocardial infarction. When a trial of effectiveness was performed, it was stopped prematurely because of the increased mortality in the test group receiving the drug. It has been estimated that more Americans died from this treatment than were killed in World War II.[10]

Another key figure in the development of EBP was Archie Cochrane (1909–1988). Cochrane became frustrated early in his career with the lack of knowledge about effective treatment. Whilst a medical prisoner of war, he related how he received a propaganda pamphlet about clinical freedom and democracy. He mused that he already had considerable clinical freedom in the camp but did not know what to use since there was no real evidence that any of the available treatments worked. A distinguished career as an epidemiologist cemented these concepts, which are presented in his classic 1971 monograph *Effectiveness and Efficiency*.[13] Writing in 1979, he stated 'It is surely a great criticism of our profession that we have not organized a critical summary, by specialty or subspecialty, updated periodically, of all relevant randomized controlled trials'.[14] Such a plea led directly to the remarkable project known as the Cochrane Collaboration, an international collective with the aim of producing high quality systematic reviews of medical (and oral health care) interventions (see Chapter 6).

The concept of what was termed 'evidence based medicine' burst into general awareness in 1992 with the publication of a paper by the clinical epidemiology group at McMaster University in Canada.[15] Their challenge was to adopt EBP since it 'de-emphasizes intuition, unsystematic clinical experience and pathophysiological rationale as sufficient grounds for clinical decision making'. Please note that the call was not to ignore these other aspects of dentistry and medicine, but rather the intent was to place increased emphasis on a systematic appraisal of the evidence. Since 1992, the concepts of EBP have spread rapidly to many fields of health care and to many different countries.

Evidence based practice and dentistry

There have been a number of important landmarks in the development of evidence based practice in dentistry. One of the first was the setting up of the Oral Health Group of the Cochrane Collaboration in 1994 by Alexia Antczak Bouckoms. Subsequently, the editorial base moved to Manchester University in 1997, with Bill Shaw and Helen Worthington as co-ordinating editors, and is described in some detail in Chapter 7. To date, the group has published nine systematic reviews in areas such as orthodontics, cancer therapy, oral medicine and periodontology and has collected more than 11,000 citations to clinical trials in dentistry.

Further fundamental contributions to the development of EBP in dentistry were made by Derek Richards and Alan Lawrence, with the publication in 1995 of a manifesto describing evidence based dentistry and the setting up of the Centre for Evidence Based Dentistry website by Derek Richards in the same year. Another group that has set out to disseminate evidence based dentistry activities is the International Evidence Based Dentistry Working Group. This group was set up by Amid Ismail and Nigel Pitts and meets at the International Association of Dental Research. Several representative bodies of dental specialities are embracing systematic review methods as the foundation for 'state of the art' workshops and the European Federation of Periodontology presented their first such workshop in 2002. The number of systematic reviews in dentistry is growing and major systematic reviews have been published by the NHS Centre for Reviews and Dissemination in York including: water fluoridation,[16] wisdom teeth removal,[17] and choosing dental restorations.[18]

The journal *Evidence-Based Dentistry* was first published in 1998 and was closely modelled on the evidence based medical journal. Each issue contains educational articles about the principles of EBP in relation to dentistry as well as quality-appraised abstracts or summaries of systematic reviews and clinical trials. Encouragingly, dental journals are becoming much more involved in evidence based activities; the *British Dental Journal* and the *Journal of Orthodontics* were the first dental journals to adopt the internationally recognized CONSORT (Consolidated Standards Of

Reporting Trials) guidelines as a standard for the reporting of clinical trials.[19,20] Other evidence based resources are listed at the end of the chapter.

Conclusions

Evidence based dentistry can help to provide clinicians with a systematic evidence base to help build decisions in practice. Evidence in isolation has little value and the skilled dentist will incorporate the results from this evidence base with an accurate assessment of the patient's problems and their preferences in reaching a solution. Focused question setting is an essential first step in this process and gets easier (and quicker) with practise. Defining the real essence of the problem is the key to good evidence based dentistry.

Acknowledgement

I am indebted to Sir Iain Chalmers at the UK Cochrane Centre for the provocative quotation by Smith which he uses in the introduction to the new edition of Archie Cochrane's classic 1971 monograph, *Effectiveness and efficiency*.[13]

EBP resources

Books
Sackett DL, Strauss SE, Richardson WS et al, *Evidence-based Medicine. How to practice and teach EBM,* 2nd edn (Churchill Livingstone: Edinburgh, 2000). Greenhalgh T, Donald A, *Evidence based health care workbook. Understanding research* (BMJ Publishing Group: London, 2000).

CD ROM
Evidence-based health care workbook and evidence-based health care CD-ROM (Update Software: Oxford, 1999).

This is an excellent package for self-directed learning and covers basic concepts, asking focused questions, finding evidence, critical appraisal and statistics made simple.

Websites

http://www.ihs.ox.ac.uk/cebd/
Centre for Evidence-Based Dentistry. An excellent collection of information and links to evidence based sites with many directly relevant to dentistry.

http://www.update-software.com/clibhome/clib.htm
The Cochrane Library, including reviews conducted by the Cochrane Collaboration and quality appraised abstracts of systematic reviews conducted by other groups. There are now nine Cochrane systematic reviews directly related to oral health and many protocols for reviews in progress.

http://www.nelh.nhs.uk/
The National Electronic Library for Health. This is a remarkable project to provide ready access to the best health information in the world. The pilot site is up and running and there is free access to much of it. Members of staff with an NHS affiliation (including dentists), are able to register for free access to the restricted areas including the Cochrane Library. There is no oral health branch library yet.

http://cebm.jr2.ox.ac.uk/
Centre for Evidence-based Medicine. Still a good site for general information about EBP.

http://www.lib.umich.edu/hw/dent/clinical/eb.html
University of Michigan Dentistry Library. Pat Anderson has put together an outstanding amount of evidence based dentistry information with access to full text articles.

http://hebw.uwcm.ac.uk/
Health Evidence Bulletins Wales. This site has a good oral health section. The information is due for updating soon.

http://www.sign.ac.uk/
Scottish Intercollegiate Guidelines Network. Two guidelines on oral health and more to come.

www.nettingtheevidence.org.uk
University of Sheffield. Probably the best collection of evidence based
links of any site.

References

1. Smith AFM, Mad cows and ecstasy: chance and choice in an evidence-based society, *J Roy Stat Soc* (1996) **159**:367–383.
2. Muir Gray JA, *Evidence-Based Healthcare*, (Churchill Livingstone: Edinburgh, 1997).
3. *Management of Unerupted and Impacted Third Molar Teeth* (SIGN Publication 43, 2000). http://www.sign.ac.uk/guidelines/fulltext/43/index.html
4. Needleman IG, Giedrys-Leeper E, Tucker RJ et al, Guided tissue regeneration for periodontal infra-bony defects (Cochrane Review). In: *The Cochrane Library*, Issue 2 (Update Software: Oxford, 2001). http://www.update-software.com/clibhome/clib.htm
5. Richardson W, Wilson M, Nishikawa J et al, The well-built clinical question: a key to evidence-based decisions, *ACP J Club* (1995) **123**: A123.
6. Richards D, Asking the right question right, *Evidence-Based Dentistry* (2000) **2**: 20–21.
7. Silagy C, Mant D, Fowler G et al, Nicotine replacement therapy for smoking cessation (Cochrane Review). In: *The Cochrane Library*, Issue 2 (Update Software: Oxford, 2001). http://www.update-software.com/clibhome/clib.htm
8. Hughes JR, Stead LF, Lancaster T, Antidepressants for smoking cessation (Cochrane Review). In: *The Cochrane Library*, Issue 2 (Update Software: Oxford, 2001). http://www.update-software.com/clibhome/clib.htm
9. The virtual office of the Surgeon General, *Tobacco Cessation Guidelines*, 2000. http://www.surgeongeneral.gov/tobacco/
10. Swales J, The troublesome search for evidence: three cultures in need of integration, *J R Soc Med* (2000) **93**:402–407.
11. Rangachari PK, Evidence-based medicine: old French wine with a new Canadian label? *J R Soc Med* (1997) **90**:280–284.
12. Mathews JR, *Quantification and The Quest for Medical Certainty*, (Princeton University Press: Princeton, 1995).
13. Cochrane AL, *Effectiveness and Efficiency: Random Reflections on Health Services*, (reissued, Royal Society of Medicine Press: London, 1999).
14. Cochrane AL, 1931–1971: a critical review, with particular reference to the medical profession. In: *Medicines for the Year 2000*, (Office of Health Economics: London, 1979.)
15. EBM Working Group, Evidence based medicine, *JAMA* (1992) **268**:2420–2425.
16. *A Systematic Review of Public Water Fluoridation* (NHS Centre for Reviews and Dissemination: York, 2000). http://www.york.ac.uk/inst/crd/fluorid.htm
17. *The Effectiveness and Cost-effectiveness of the Prophylactic Removal of Wisdom Teeth and Wisdom Teeth Removal* (NHS R&D Health Technology Assessment Programme, 2000). http://www.hta.nhsweb.nhs.uk/htapubs.htm

18. *Dental Restorations: What Type of Filling?* (NHS Centre for Reviews and Dissemination, 1999). http://www.york.ac.uk/inst/crd/ehc52.htm
19. Needleman IG, CONSORT, *Br Dent J* (1999) **186**:207.
20. Consort statement website. http://www.consort-statement.org/

chapter 2

Different types of evidence: where and how to find them

Jayne E Harrison and Sylvia R Bickley

In this chapter we will be describing the different research methods that you are likely to find reported in the dental literature and also giving guidance on the strength of this evidence. We will then provide pointers as to where this evidence can be found and how it can be accessed, together with an indication of some of the problems that you might encounter when searching the literature.

Research methods

The research methods used in a study will depend on what question it is addressing. For any given clinical question some research designs will provide information that is more valid than others (Table 2.1).[1,2] Before assessing the strength of evidence provided by studies using different research methods, we will give a brief description of the main research methods that are used in clinical research, together with examples of papers where each method has been used.

Hierarchy of evidence

For assessments of therapeutic interventions, well-designed randomized controlled trials (RCTs), confirming the same hypothesis, have for many

Table 2.1 Guidelines for selecting articles that are most likely to provide valid results for a given clinical question

Question	Most appropriate research method	Key questions
Therapy	Clinical trial	Was the allocation of treatments to patients randomized?
		Were the patients, clinicians and/or assessors blind to treatment allocation?
		Were all the patients who entered the trial accounted for and attributed at its conclusion?
Diagnosis or screening	Cross-sectional survey	Was there an independent, blind comparison with a reference standard?
		Did the patient sample include an appropriate range of the sort of patients to whom the diagnostic/screening test will be applied in clinical practice?
Prognosis	Cohort study	Was there a representative patient sample, at a well-defined point in their disease?
		Was the follow-up sufficiently long and complete?
Causation	Case–control or cohort study	Were there clearly identified comparison groups that were similar with respect to important determinants of the outcome of interest?
		Were outcomes and exposures measured in the same way in the groups being compared?
Summary of evidence	Systematic review	Did the review address a focused clinical question?
		Were the criteria used to select articles for inclusion appropriate?

Modified from Oxman et al[1] and Greenhalgh[2]

Anecdotal case report
Cross-sectional   survey
Case series without a control
Case–control observational study
Cohort study with a literature control
Analyses using computer databases
Cohort study with a historical control group
Unconfirmed randomized controlled clinical trial
Confirmed definitive randomized controlled clinical trials
Systematic review of randomized controlled clinical trials

Figure 2.1 *Hierarchy of evidence.*

years been recognized as providing the strongest level of evidence on which to base our clinical decisions.[3,4] However, with the development of systematic review and meta-analytic techniques, we can now see systematic reviews as the foundation stone of our pyramidal hierarchy of evidence (Figure 2.1).[2,5–8] Although considerable weight is placed on the evidence from RCTs and systematic reviews of RCTs, these research methods are not appropriate to answer every question. It must be remembered that valuable information can be obtained from other levels of evidence and each has its role to play in providing evidence about the treatment we provide for our patients (Table 2.1). We have presented the key features of the main research designs used in clinical dental research, together with examples of papers where they have been used, in Table 2.2.

Finding the evidence

Having asked questions related to our patients' problems, where and how do we find the evidence to answer them? We can ask a friend or colleague, but do they know any better than us what the answer is, and from what angle are they approaching the problem? We can check the papers in our filing cabinet, but how many papers do each of us keep?

Table 2.2 The key features and examples of different research methods

Research method		Key features	Examples
Clinical trial		Assesses whether one healthcare intervention is better than another, a placebo or no treatment. Is prospective and controlled. Allocation to test/control groups is pre-determined.	Competing posterior composites;[9] antibiotic vs placebo,[10] no lingual nerve retraction.[11]
	Random	Allocation to patient/quadrant/tooth according to a sequence generated from a table of random numbers or its electronic equivalent. Minimizes risk of all forms of bias.	Random allocation of patients to have treatment or no treatment.[12]
	Quasi-random	Allocation to alternate patients or according to date of birth, case note number, day of week, side of mouth, quadrant. Prone to allocation bias.	Allocation of different interventions to a specific quadrant.[13]
	Haphazard	A group of patients is divided into groups. Prone to allocation bias.	Three brands of composites used in 33 patients.[9]

Table 2.2 Continued

Research method		Key features	Examples
Cohort Study		Describes what happens to patients without actively intervening with the treatment they receive. Can be prospective or retrospective. May have a separate control group or be uncontrolled.	Treatment outcomes of fixed or removable implant supported prosthesis.[14] Approximal caries prevalence and caries progression in the late teens.[15]
	Uncontrolled	An uncontrolled cohort study describing the outcome of treatment for a group of patients.	Alveolar bone grafting for children with cleft palate.[16] Implant survival in 440 patients after 7 years.[17]
	Case series	A small case series describing the outcome of treatment of a few (< 5–10) cases or reporting potential problems with treatment.	Outcome of treatment with a new appliance.[18] Complications of tongue piercing.[19]
	Case report		

Table 2.2 Continued

Research method		Key features	Examples
Controlled	Literature	Comparison made to information on patients in a published paper or growth study. Prone to chronological and/or geographical bias.	Comparison made to values calculated from several published studies.[20]
	Historical	Comparison made with patients treated previously in the same unit/place. Prone to chronological bias.	Caries in the primary dentition following the discontinuation of water fluoridation.[21]
	Matched	Comparison made with patients who are similar in respect to one or two specific criteria. Prone to allocation bias.	Pairs of children matched for socio-demographic criteria.[22]
	Concurrent	Control group treated at the same time as the study group. Prone to allocation bias.	Patients treated at the same time but with different restorative materials.[23]
Survey		Describes how things are now. Sample may include all or a random sample of the population of interest. Does not usually have a separate control group but internal comparisons can be made.	Perception of the impact of dental health on the quality of life in people from different socio-economic backgrounds.[24]
Cross-sectional		Data collected from sample members on one occasion by questionnaire or clinical examination	Management of the primary carious lesions.[25] Prevalence of orthodontic treatment need.[26]
Longitudinal		Data collected from sample members on two or more occasions.	Changes in periodontal bone height in an adult population over a period of 17 years.[27]

Table 2.2 Continued

Research method		Key features	Examples
Case–control study		Asks what makes a group of individuals different with respect to treatment received or environmental factors. Retrospective and look back in time.	Factors influencing root resorption following fixed appliance treatment[28] Acidic dietary factors associated with erosion.[29]
	Multi-variant methods	Identify factors that have a significant influence on the outcome of interest.	Factors associated with the length of orthodontic treatment.[30] Smoking habits as risk factors for periodontal disease and tooth loss.[31]
Review article		Summarizes information from several previously published papers on a specific topic.	
	Narrative review	Based on haphazard selection of papers related to the subject of the review.	Tooth wear.[32]
	Systematic review	Papers are identified, critically appraised and the results synthesized according to a defined protocol.	Prevention of oral lesions for patients being treated for cancer.[33]
	Meta-analysis	Combines the results from several different clinical trials to obtain an overall estimate of the effectiveness of a particular intervention.	Orthodontic treatment for posterior crossbites.[34] Systemic tetracycline in chronic adult periodontitis.[35]

How old are the papers and why have we kept or copied those ones in the first place? We can then extend our search into the wider world of published information, whether in the form of a textbook or review article found in the library, electronically, via the Internet or by hand searching key journals.

The literature

In our rapidly changing world, we are suffering from information overload. Every year over 2 million articles are published in 20,000 biomedical journals of which about 700 are related to dentistry.[36,37] It is impossible for any one clinician to keep on top of all this published information let alone the work that remains unpublished. Bias exists as to which studies get published and where they get published.[38,39] Therefore we have to ask 'Why haven't they got published?' and 'Why have they been published in that journal?' Are unpublished studies less valid or less relevant? Have they been rejected from journals? Do investigators or journal editors think the results are uninteresting? Have the investigators lost interest, run out of the energy required, or no longer need to get their work published? Higher impact journals, in dentistry (and medicine) tend to be published in English,[37] so does writing a scientific paper in a language that is not the investigators' first language act as a real barrier to publication in these journals? Evidence in the medical literature suggests that there is no difference in the quality of trials reported in non-English language journals,[40] so should we disregard the results of a study because it is published in French, Spanish or Chinese? Have these studies been rejected by English language journals? Are the results only applicable to a specific population? Just as bias exists in what gets published and where it gets published, it is likely that bias exists in which studies get read, if only in relation to which journal(s) drop through our letterboxes correspondent to the dental societies to which we belong.

The need to identify and bring together valid and clinically useful articles from a large number of journals has led to the publication of several evidence based 'secondary' journals. Surprisingly these journals are relatively thin and are published infrequently. The first of these (*ACP*

Journal Club) appeared in 1991. It was followed by *Evidence-Based Medicine* in 1995 and in 1998 *Evidence-Based Dentistry* (EBD) was published as a supplement to the *British Dental Journal*; this has now become a journal in its own right. These journals aim to screen relevant journals for good, useful evidence on topics applicable to their areas of interest. The papers are then critically assessed with respect to methods used, results obtained and whether the conclusions drawn can be supported. EBD also includes a commentary that places papers in their clinical perspective, highlighting how and where they are relevant to clinical practice and whether practice should continue or change as a result of the findings.[41]

Textbooks and literature reviews

Textbooks and literature reviews often cover a broad range of issues related to a particular subject. They can only be as up to date as their most recent reference and therefore go out of date quickly, sometimes even before they are published. Textbooks and reviews do not usually specify a literature search strategy, with papers being selected, assessed and summarized haphazardly rather than by using a comprehensive, systematic search strategy, critically appraising all the available evidence and synthesizing the data in a quantitative way. Consequently recommendations contained in textbooks and traditional reviews may lag behind by more than a decade, endorsing an effective treatment or continuing to advocate a therapy long after it has been shown to be ineffective or even harmful.[42]

Systematic reviews

Systematic reviews bring together large amounts of information from as many published and unpublished clinical trials as possible and analyze the data in a process called meta-analysis.[43] This relatively new scientific activity has evolved to produce systematic reviews that separate insignificant, unsound or redundant research in the literature from the salient and critical studies that are worthy of further consideration.[44]

Systematic reviews are prepared as methodically and carefully as a piece of primary research. Initially a protocol is written that describes which trials will be included and how they will be identified, selected and evaluated. These reviews may include a meta-analysis of the results of several trials if this is appropriate, and the editorial process ensures that they are checked and verified for validity and clinical relevance. Antman and colleagues examined the differences between traditional and systematic reviews.[42] They compared the recommendations of clinical experts writing review articles and textbook chapters with the results of meta-analyses of randomized controlled trials of treatments for myocardial infarction. They found that there were discrepancies between the results of meta-analyses and the recommendations of expert reviewers. Review articles often failed to mention important advances in effective interventions. In some cases, treatment that had been shown to have no effect on mortality, or was potentially harmful, continued to be recommended by several clinical experts in reviews and textbooks.

Electronic databases

The availability of electronic databases as accessible sources of evidence is increasing rapidly. There are two types of electronic database. The first is bibliographic and lists primary research e.g. MEDLINE, EMBASE. The second type consists of databases that take the user directly to primary or secondary publications of relevant clinical evidence e.g. the Cochrane Database of Systematic Reviews (see below).

The largest and most readily available electronic database is MEDLINE. It is produced by the United States National Library of Medicine and contains more than 11 million citations that date back to 1966. It became available to clinical users in the 1980s and since 1997 it has been available free of charge on the Internet through the PubMed website http://www.ncbi.nlm.nih.gov/PubMed. However, the journals included on the MEDLINE database are biased towards English language journals and especially American ones. The European equivalent of MEDLINE is EMBASE, a database produced in the Netherlands by Elsevier Science. It has a strong European and pharmacological content, and some overlap with MEDLINE in terms of the journals covered. Unfortunately, user costs are higher than MEDLINE as there is no free version and it is not as widely available.[45] Most postgraduate centres, hospital and university libraries will have an institutional subscription to one or more of these sources. Most clinicians will be able to gain access to these and other specialized databases via their affiliated education centres.

Searching electronic databases appears to be a very attractive way of tracking down relevant trials, but unfortunately even the most experienced searchers will only identify about half of the available relevant trials on a topic.[46] This is very disappointing, especially as most of the missed citations are in fact in the databases. The main reasons why these citations are not picked up lies in the indexing of the literature that is based on descriptors used in the paper. Lack of detail in the paper will affect the quality of indexing and ultimately the quality and results of a search. One way of increasing the retrieval of relevant articles is for journals to use structured abstracts, where the author systematically discloses the objective, design, setting, subject, interventions, outcomes, results and conclusions of a study.[8,47,48] These are now being used by an increasing number of journals and are one of the recommendations of the CONSORT guidelines.[49] With increasing numbers of journals using structured abstracts and accepting these guidelines, it is hoped that the quality of the yield from searches of electronic databases will improve in the future.

Hand searching

For earlier publications, 'hand searching' journals, which involves searching journals page by page, is probably the best way of tracing as many relevant articles as possible. Recognizing the importance of identifying randomized controlled trials to systematic reviewing, the Cochrane Collaboration set up a worldwide journals hand searching program to identify RCTs and Controlled Clinical Trials (CCTs). This highly organized programme, co-ordinated by the New England Cochrane Center, Providence Office, avoids duplication of effort and provides access to trials found only by hand searching through the Cochrane Controlled Trials Register in the Cochrane Library. The master list of journals being searched can be accessed via http://www.cochrane.us.

From the aforementioned it will be seen that no single source can be relied upon to provide all the evidence and that literature searches need to be approached in a systematic way. The following section will introduce the reader to the basic rules that must be applied for effective searching, and by presenting a worked example provide guidance on building a search strategy.

Electronic literature searching

Before starting to search, time spent identifying appropriate search terms and building these into a structured search strategy will be time well spent. The aim of the search strategy should be a balance between sensitivity, i.e. a search wide enough to guard against missing relevant articles, but which will inevitably retrieve some non-relevant articles, and specificity, i.e. a search so closely focused to the subject that it may exclude relevant articles. In the identification of RCTs for systematic reviews the sensitivity of the search will be paramount.

Proficiency in searching is an art that can only be learned through practice and gaining knowledge and understanding of the rules that must be applied to searching individual databases. Information and guidance on this is usually available from medical libraries, or database providers' points of access (e.g. NLM PubMed, Ovid, Silver Platter, etc) via Internet web sites, or directly from the database help files. For the busy clinician, however, it is advisable to obtain the guidance of a medical librarian or information specialist. Their expertise in literature searching combined with the clinician's subject knowledge will provide the complementary skills needed to build the most appropriate and effective search strategy.

Identifying search terms

Search terms should include controlled vocabulary and free-text terms.

Controlled vocabulary refers to the subject headings (indexing terms) that are used in electronic databases. Some databases, such as MEDLINE, EMBASE and CINAHL, use subject headings that are arranged in a hierarchically structured format like the branches of a tree, with broader concepts near the top and more specific terms lower down. In MEDLINE this is called the MeSH Tree (MeSH® standing for 'medical subject headings') and in EMBASE – EMTREE. Other databases may use a structured thesaurus of concepts arranged alphabetically. Using the hierarchically structured trees or thesauri enables searchers to broaden or narrow their search. Searchers will find the NLM's MeSH browser, which has full details of MeSH terms, their indexing and hierarchy, a valuable resource. You will find this at Internet site www.nlm.nih.gov/mesh/MBrowser. html or in hard copy in the reference section of medical libraries.

The section of the MeSH tree presented in Figure 2.2 shows a dental example where the broadest subject heading is orthodontics, with more specific headings in the branches below. Any point in the hierarchy can be searched to include the terms beneath it by applying the 'explode' function in the database's search engine. For example, linking the instruction 'explode' to the term 'orthodontics' would automatically include all of the search terms presented in the orthodontic hierarchy

Orthodontics
    Orthodontic-appliance-design
    Orthodontic appliances
        Occlusal-splints
        Orthodontic-appliances-functional
            Activator-appliances
        Orthodontic-appliances-removable
            Activator-appliances
            Extraoral-traction-appliances
        Orthodontic-brackets
        Orthodontic-retainers
        Orthodontic-wires
    Orthodontics-corrective
        Occlusal-adjustment
        Orthodontic-space-closure
        Palatal-expansion-technique
        Tooth-movement
    Orthodontics-interceptive
        Serial-extraction
    Orthodontics-preventive
        Space-maintenance

Figure 2.2 *Section of MeSH tree showing hierarchically structured format.*

below. Alternatively we could focus the search to a specific area of interest within orthodontics by applying the 'explode' function to a branch lower down the tree. For example, applying 'explode in this tree' to the subject heading 'orthodontic-appliances-functional' would focus the search to only retrieve articles indexed with the terms 'orthodontic-appliances-functional 'or' activator-appliances'.

Subject headings (controlled vocabulary) are assigned in accordance with their importance to the subject of an article by experienced indexers. Terms from controlled vocabulary will only be searched for in the dedicated indexing field, whereas free-text terms can be searched for anywhere in the record. Confining the search to one or the other will affect the search in a number of ways. For example, if using only controlled vocabulary, only the exact indexing term (unless it has been 'exploded') will be searched for in the indexing field. You should also be aware when searching PubMed that new records are added daily in advance of being indexed. At this stage retrieval of these records will be dependent on the free-text terms in your search strategy. Furthermore, some databases (e.g. the Cochrane Controlled Trials Register) are compiled from a range of sources and their records may not all be indexed in the same way.

Using free-text might appear to be a 'catch all' option, but the search will be confined to finding the exact match of those text word(s) in the title, abstract or keywords of the electronic record. It will also miss things that exploded indexing will pick up. For example take the term 'periodontitis', when used as free-text this will only pick up articles where this exact term appears. The same word used as an exploded MeSH term will pick up not only articles where this term appears, but also articles containing the subordinate terms beneath it in the MeSH tree:

Periodontitis	{Subject heading exploded}
Periodontal-abscess	Subordinate
Periodontal-pocket	terms in the
Periodontitis-juvenile	MeSH tree

Whilst in general, using only controlled vocabulary may restrict retrieval of relevant records, using free-text only is more likely to produce many non-relevant records.

The searcher should be aware that controlled vocabulary and free-text may also be expressed or spelled differently as MeSH terms use American spellings. A dental example would be 'apicectomy' in free-text and 'API-COECTOMY' as a MeSH controlled vocabulary term; or 'anaesthetics' (free-text) and 'ANESTHETICS' (controlled vocabulary). Another example would be 'topical fluoride', which is how the phrase is likely to be expressed as free-text, but is indexed as 'FLUORIDES-TOPICAL' in MeSH.

Truncations and operators

An understanding of how results can be affected by the way free-text terms are presented will help refine the search. 'Truncation' symbols inserted at the end of a free-text word will expand the search to retrieve all possible suffix variations of the word. An example would be the truncation symbol (asterisk) in 'topical fluoride*' which will retrieve articles containing either the phrase 'topical fluoride' or 'topical fluorides'.

A comprehensive search strategy will include both controlled vocabulary and free-text terms linked systematically by appropriate search operators. Operators are words used to link search terms, such as 'AND' 'OR' 'NEAR' 'NEXT' etc. The operator AND is used when the paper must contain both search terms. In Figure 2.3(a), papers containing both terms ('child*' AND 'topical fluoride') are retrieved where the circles overlap.

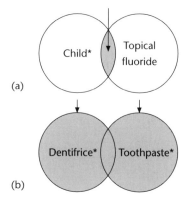

Figure 2.3 *The effect of linking search items with the operators (a) 'AND' or (b) 'OR'. In (a) (child* AND topical fluoride) only papers containing both terms will be retrieved. In (b) (toothpaste* OR dentifrice*) papers containing either term will be retrieved.*

The operator OR is used when a paper may contain either search term. In Figure 2.3(b) any papers containing the word 'dentifrice(s)' OR 'toothpaste(s)' will be retrieved.

Inserting the operator NEXT between terms will retrieve articles where the terms are adjacent to each other; for example oral NEXT surgery. Using the operator AND in this same example would also retrieve all the articles containing the phrase 'oral surgery' but because the words 'oral' and surgery' can be anywhere in the article, this search is likely to pick up many non-relevant articles. Consider, for example, an abstract that reads 'Oral antibiotics were administered prior to the orthopaedic surgery'.

It should be noted that operators that control proximity of search terms (e.g. NEXT or NEAR) might be used or expressed differently depending on which resource provider you use. For example, some search interfaces (e.g. Ovid) use the letters ADJ (for adjacent) in place of 'NEXT'. A number placed immediately after the letters ADJ (e.g. 'restorations ADJ4 molars') will allow the search to find papers containing both terms, so long as they are within the indicated number of words (in this example, 4) of each other (e.g. 'restorations involving molars', 'restorations in primary molars'). Particular attention should be paid to the search rules that apply to proximity searching, since their use in some databases is not as flexible as in others.

Subject headings in different databases

It is important to note that subject headings identified for one database may not be applicable in another. For this reason, controlled vocabulary in search strategies needs to be tailored to each database, but once you have built your search strategy it will be fairly straightforward to revise it for a different database. Similarly, operators and symbols may be different depending on the resource provider: for example the symbol for truncation in PubMed is an asterisk (*), in Ovid it is a dollar sign ($). Before starting to search, familiarizing yourself with the rules that apply to the particular resource you are using will save a lot of time and frustration later.

Choosing the best resource for your needs

Most questions associated with applying evidence based dentistry to clinical dentistry will revolve around the effectiveness of competing interventions that are provided for patients. To answer these questions, up-to-date systematic reviews of randomized controlled trials (RCTs) are generally accepted as being the most reliable source of evidence. The best place to search for systematic reviews of RCTs is the Cochrane Library, which is made up of a collection of electronic databases including the Cochrane Database of Systematic Reviews and the Database of Abstracts of Reviews of Effectiveness. If there are no relevant up-to-date systematic reviews in your area of interest, you should consider evidence contained in the individual reports of RCTs. The Cochrane Controlled Trials Register (CCTR), also available in the Cochrane Library, is recognized as being the best single source of such reports.[50] The CCTR is the result of a number of ongoing projects within the Cochrane Collaboration worldwide[51] and brings together in one bibliographic database, citations to controlled clinical trials from across the world (Issue 3, 2002 contained 348,740 citations). Updated quarterly, it is sourced from searching electronic databases, including MEDLINE and other major healthcare databases, conference proceedings and trials found only through the Cochrane Collaboration's worldwide journal hand searching program.

The Cochrane Library is available through many university libraries, postgraduate medical centres and some local libraries. It is also available through personal subscription on CD – a yearly subscription covers four quarterly issues. (Details available from Update Software Ltd, Oxford, or Update Software Inc, Vista, CA, USA or via websites www.cochranelibrary.com and www.update-software.com.)

From September 2002 respective government funding enabled anyone in England, Wales and Ireland with access to the Internet to connect to the Cochrane Library free of charge. This initiative was one in a series of steps aimed at making the Cochrane Library readily accessible throughout the world. A list of all the countries which currently have a national provision in place for access to the Cochrane Library can be found on the Update Software website at www.update-software.com/clibng/usernotfound/showcountries.asp.

Searching to answer a research question

As an example let us take as our research question: 'Are fissure sealants effective for preventing dental caries?' and start our search with the Cochrane Controlled Trials Register (CCTR). First we need to identify the sections of the question as:

1. The population (children)
2. The intervention (fissure sealants)
3. The outcome (prevention of dental caries and enamel decalcification)

A structured search strategy will be more controllable and easier to check for inclusions and omissions than a haphazard list of search terms and the best approach is to use the section headings to form the structure on which the search strategy will be built. Be aware however, that when sensitivity is important, it is probably best to base the search framework on two section headings – in this example, 'intervention' and 'outcome'. This is because the terms in each separate section will first be 'OR'd together and then the results from each section will be linked with the operator 'AND'. At this stage at least one term from each section must appear in the electronic record for the reference to be retrieved. Consequently the more sections introduced, the greater the chance of 'losing' some relevant papers, especially where the electronic record may only have a title and keywords on which to search.

Start by considering which terms might be included and list these under the appropriate heading, keeping controlled vocabulary (identified in Figure 2.4 by upper case text) and free-text terms (lower case) separate. The Cochrane Library contains the MEDLINE MeSH thesaurus which conveniently enables the searcher to select controlled vocabulary and build it directly into the search strategy. Under each of the headings a range of possible search terms will be listed, using a combination of controlled vocabulary and free-text terms as given in Figure 2.4.

Keeping the concept of group headings, the next stage is to link the terms and build them into a search strategy (Figure 2.5).

Building well thought out search strategies takes concentration and is time consuming. Fortunately most database providers enable you to save

INTERVENTION	OUTCOME
PIT AND FISSURE SEALANTS (ME)	(Explode) TOOTH DEMINERALIZATION (ME)
RESIN CEMENTS (ME)	DMF-INDEX (ME)
GLASS IONOMER CEMENTS (ME)	dmf* NEXT index
Tooth NEAR seal*	DMF* NEXT index
Teeth NEAR seal*	'dental caries' NEAR prevent*
Fissure NEAR seal*	'dental decay' NEAR prevent*
Resin NEAR seal*	'dental caries' NEAR control*
Resin NEAR cement*	'dental decay' NEAR control*
Dental NEAR seal*	dental NEXT decay
Glass NEXT ionomer*	Tooth NEXT decay*
	Teeth NEXT decay*
	Decalcif* NEAR tooth
	Decalcif* NEAR teeth
	Decalcif* NEAR enamel*
	demineralli* NEAR tooth
	Demineralli* NEAR teeth
	Demineralli* NEAR enamel*
	evaluat*
	effective*

***Figure 2.4**. Identifying search terms.*
(ME) = MeSH terms (controlled vocabulary)

your search strategy so that, once built, you can recall it at any time. It is also good advice to save your search strategy at intervals as you build it, so that if you make a mistake you can recall your last save rather than having to start from the beginning.

In the example in Figure 2.4 it will be seen that to protect the sensitiv-

```
#1      (Explode) PIT AND FISSURE SEALANTS [99]
#2      fissure NEAR seal* [203]
#3      (Explode) GLASS-IONOMER-CEMENTS [183]
#4      RESIN CEMENTS [99]
#5      resin* NEAR cement* [209]
#6      resin* NEAR seal*) [68]
#7      glass NEXT ionomer* [275]
#8      dental NEAR seal* [94]
#9      tooth NEAR seal* [32]
#10     teeth NEAR seal* [81]
#11     fissure* NEAR seal* [203]
#12     #3 OR #4 OR #5 OR #6 OR #7 [411]
#13     #8 OR #9 OR #10 OR #11 [251]
#14     #12 AND #13 [77]
#15     #1 OR #2 OR #14 [215]
#16     TOOTH REMINERALIZATION [54]
#17     (Explode) TOOTH DEMINERALIZATION [561]
#18     dental NEXT caries [952]
#19     dental NEXT decay [18]
#20     decalcif* NEAR tooth [2]
#21     decalcif* NEAR teeth [11]
#22     decalcif* NEAR enamel [9]
#23     deminerali* NEAR tooth [74]
#24     deminerali* NEAR teeth [14]
#25     deminerali* NEAR enamel [64]
#26     reminerali* NEAR tooth [77]
#27     reminerali* NEAR teeth [3]
#28     reminerali* NEAR enamel [56]
#29     recalcif* NEAR tooth [0]
#30     recalcif* NEAR teeth [0]
#31     recalcif* NEAR enamel [0]
#32     DMF-INDEX [208]
#33     DMF* NEXT index [348]
#34     DMF* NEXT indices) [2]
#35     caries NEAR prevent* [678]
#36     decay NEAR prevent* [22]
#37     caries NEAR control* [633]
#38     decay NEAR control* [25]
#39     #35 OR #36 OR #37 OR #38 AND dental [687]
#40     effective* OR evaluat* [125952]
#41     #16 OR #17 OR #18 OR #19 OR #20 OR #21 OR #22 OR #23 OR #24 OR #25 OR
        #26 OR #27 OR #28 OR #29 OR #30 OR #31 OR #32 OR #33 OR #34 OR #39 OR
        #40[126603]
#42     #15 AND #41 [173]
```

Figure 2.5 *The structured search strategy.*
(ME) = MeSH terms (controlled vocabulary); MeSH terms are shown in upper case; free-text in lower case. Operators are shown in bold upper case. The Cochrane Library's search engine includes the operator 'NEAR' which retrieves papers where the words linked by this operator appear within six words of each other. Terms in parenthesis will be automatically executed first by the search engine. As each line of the search is executed the number of 'hits' will be shown in square brackets as shown above. This example shows the number of records retrieved from the CENTRAL/CCTR database in the Cochrane Library, Issue 2, 2002. As the searches from each group are combined it can be seen how the record retrieval becomes more focused to the subject of the research question: at search line 42, the intervention terms have been combined with the outcome terms, giving a total of 173 records retrieved.

Note: As the Cochrane Library search engine is not case sensitive #33 and #34 will pick up both DMF*or dmf* index.

ity of the search, only two of the three elements of the research question have been developed into the search strategy, with each of the elements being searched separately before linking the chosen search terms with the operator 'OR'. The combined result from each of the groups is then linked with the Boolean[4] operator 'AND' to focus the search to retrieve only those articles that contain terms from both the intervention and the outcome elements of our research question (Figure 2.5). The articles retrieved should be examined to identify any other relevant search terms that may need to be incorporated into a revised search strategy.

In this part of the chapter, we have endeavoured to give the reader an insight into approaching a literature search systematically. It will be seen that effective searching needs concentrated effort, a knowledge and understanding of the many facets and anomalies of searching and practice. Where accuracy of searching is paramount, the reader with limited experience is advised to seek the guidance of a medical librarian or information specialist.

Acknowledgement

The authors wish to acknowledge the contribution of Carol Lefebvre, Information Specialist at the UK Cochrane Centre, for reading an earlier draft of the section on literature searching in this chapter and for her helpful comments.

References

1. Oxman AD, Sackett DL, Guyatt GH, Users' guide to the medical literature: 1. How to get started, *JAMA* (1993) **270**:2093–2095.
2. Greenhalgh T, *How to Read a Paper: The Basis of Evidence Based Medicine* (BMJ Publishing Group: London, 1997).
3. Green SB, Byar DP, Using observational data from registries to compare treatments: the fallacy of omnimetrics, *Stat Med* (1984) 3:361–373.
4. O'Brien K, Craven R, Pitfalls in orthodontic health service research, *Br J Orthod* (1995) **22**:353–356.
5. Antczak-Bouckoms A, The anatomy of clinical research, *Clin Orthod Res* (1998) 1:75–79.

6. Deeks JD, Sheldon TA, Guidelines for undertaking systematic reviews of effectiveness. Version 4, *York Centre for Reviews and Dissemination* (1995) 35–42.
7. Guyatt GH, Sackett DL, Sinclair JC et al, Users' guides to the medical literature. IX. A method for grading health care recommendations. Evidence Based Medicine Working Group, *JAMA* (1995) **274**:1800–1804.
8. Harrison JE, Ashby D, Lennon MA, An analysis of papers published in the British and European Journals of Orthodontics, *Br J Orthod* (1996) **23**:203–209.
9. Turkun LS, Aktener BO, Twenty-four-month clinical evaluation of different posterior composite resin materials, *J Am Dent Assoc* (2001) **132**:196–203; quiz 224–225.
10. Nagle D, Reader A, Beck M et al, Effect of systemic penicillin on pain in untreated irreversible pulpitis, *Oral Surg Oral Med Oral Pathol Oral Radiol Endod* (2000) **90**:636–640.
11. Gargallo-Albiol J, Buenechea-Imaz R, Gay-Escoda C, Lingual nerve protection during surgical removal of lower third molars. A prospective randomized study, *Intl J Oral Maxillofac Surg* (2000) **29**:268–271.
12. Harradine NW, Pearson MH, Toth B, The effect of extraction of third molars on late lower incisor crowding: a randomized controlled trial, *Br J Orthod* (1998) **25**:117–122.
13. Erverdi N, Koyuturk O, Kucukkeles N, Nickel-titanium coil springs and repelling magnets: a comparison of two different intra-oral molar distalisation techniques, *Br J Orthod* (1997) **24**:47–53.
14. Zitzmann NU, Marinello CP, Treatment outcomes of fixed or removable implant-supported prostheses in the edentulous maxilla. Part I: patients' assessments, *J Prosthet Dent* (2000) **83**:424–433.
15. Hintze H, Approximal caries prevalence in Danish recruits and progression of caries in the late teens: a retrospective radiographic study, *Caries Res* (2001) **35**:27–35.
16. Boyne PJ, Sands NR, Secondary bone grafting of residual alveolar and palatal clefts, *J Oral Surg* (1972) **30**:87–92.
17. Brocard D, Barthet P, Baysse E et al, A multicenter report on 1,022 consecutively placed ITI implants: a 7-year longitudinal study, *Intl J Oral Maxillofac Implants* (2000) **15**:691–700.
18. Harrison JE, Early experiences with the Tip-Edge appliance, *Br J Orthod* (1998) **25**:1–9.
19. Perkins CS, Meisner J, Harrison JM, A complication of tongue piercing, *Br Dent J* (1997) **182**:147–148.
20. Stucki N, Ingervall B, The use of the Jasper Jumper for the correction of Class II malocclusion in the young permanent dentition, *Eur J Orthod* (1998) **20**:271–281.
21. Seppa L, Karkkainen S, Hausen H, Caries in the primary dentition, after discontinuation of water fluoridation, among children receiving comprehensive dental care, *Community Dent Oral Epidemiol* (2000) **28**:281–288.
22. Hiller KA, Wilfart G, Schmalz G, Developmental enamel defects in children with different fluoride supplementation – a follow-up study, *Caries Res* (1998) **32**:405–411.
23. Fuks AB, Araujo FB, Osorio LB et al, Clinical and radiographic assessment of

Class II esthetic restorations in primary molars, *Pediatr Dent* (2000) 22(6):479–485.

24. Grath CM, Bedi R, Gilthorpe MS, Oral health related quality of life – views of the public in the United Kingdom, *Community Dent Health* (2000) 17:3–7.

25. Sundberg H, Mejare I, Espelid I et al, Swedish dentists' decisions on preparation techniques and restorative materials, *Acta Odontol Scand* (2000) 58:135–141.

26. Holmes A, The prevalence of orthodontic treatment need, *Br J Orthod* (1992) 19:177–182.

27. Hugoson A, Laurell L, A prospective longitudinal study on periodontal bone height changes in a Swedish population, *J Clin Periodontol* (2000) 27:665–674.

28. Kaley J, Phillips C, Factors related to root resorption in edgewise practice, *Angle Orthod* (1991) 61:125–132.

29. O'Sullivan EA, Curzon ME, A comparison of acidic dietary factors in children with and without dental erosion, *ASDC J Dent Child* (2000) 67:186–192, 160.

30. Turbill EA, Richmond S, Wright JL, The time-factor in orthodontics: what influences the duration of treatments in National Health Service practices? *Community Dent Oral Epidemiol* (2001) 29:62–72.

31. Albandar JM, Streckfus CF, Adesanya MR et al, Cigar, pipe, and cigarette smoking as risk factors for periodontal disease and tooth loss, *J Periodontol* (2000) 71:1874–1881.

32. Smith BG, Bartlett DW, Robb ND, The prevalence, etiology and management of tooth wear in the United Kingdom, *J Prosthet Dent* (1997) 78:367–372.

33. Clarkson JE, Worthington HV, Eden OB, Prevention of oral mucositis or oral candidiasis for patients with cancer receiving chemotherapy (excluding head and neck cancer), Cochrane Database Syst Rev (2000) 2:CD000978

34. Harrison JE, Ashby D, Orthodontic treatment for posterior crossbites (Cochrane Review), Cochrane Database Syst Rev (2001) 1:CD000979

35. Hayes C, Antczak-Bouckoms A, Burdick E, Quality assessment and meta-analysis of systemic tetracycline use in chronic adult periodontitis, *J Clin Periodontol* (1992) 19:164–168.

36. Richards D, Lawrence A, Evidence based dentistry, *Br Dent J* (1995) 179: 270–273.

37. Richards D, Which journal should you read to keep up to date? *Evidence-Based Dentistry* (1998) 1:22–25.

38. Easterbrook PJ, Berlin JA, Gopalan R et al, Publication bias in clinical research, *Lancet* (1991) 337:867–872.

39. Dickersin K, Min YI, Meinert CL, Factors influencing publication of research results. Follow-up of applications submitted to two institutional review boards, *JAMA* (1992) 267:374–378.

40. Moher D, Fortin P, Jadad AR et al, Completeness of reporting of trials published in languages other than English: implications for conduct and reporting of systematic reviews, *Lancet* (1996) 347:363–366.

41. Lawrence A, Welcome to evidence-based dentistry *Evidence-Based Dentistry,* (1998) 1:2–3.

42. Antman EM, Lau J, Kupelnick B et al, A comparison of results of meta-analyses of randomized control trials and recommendations of clinical experts. Treatments for myocardial infarction, *JAMA* (1992) 268:240–248.

43. Mulrow CD, Rationale for systematic reviews, *BMJ* (1994) 309:597–599.

44. Morgan PP, Review articles: 2. The literature jungle, *CMAJ* (1986) **134**:98–99.
45. Hunt DL, McKibbon KA, Locating and appraising systematic reviews, *Ann Intern Med* (1997) **126**:532–538.
46. Dickersin K, Scherer R, Lefebvre C, Identifying relevant studies for systematic reviews, *BMJ* (1994) **309**:1286–1291.
47. Haynes RB, Mulrow CD, Huith EJ et al, More informative abstracts revisited, *Ann Intern Med* (1990) **113**:69–76.
48. Ad Hoc Working Group for Critical Appraisal of the Medical Literature, A proposal for more informative abstracts of clinical articles, *Ann Intern Med* (1987) **106**:598–604.
49. Moher D, Schulz KF, Altman D, The CONSORT statement: revised recommendations for improving the quality of reports of parallel-group randomised trials, *JAMA* (2001) **285**:1987–1991. Also at www.consort-statement.org/revisedstatement.htm.
50. Egger M, Davey-Smith G, Meta-analysis bias in location and selection of studies, *BMJ* (1998) **316**:61–66.
51. Lefebvre C, Clarke MJ, Identifying randomised trials. In: Egger M, Davey-Smith G, Altman DA, eds *Systematic Reviews in Health Care: Meta-analysis in Context*, 2nd edn (BMJ Publishing Group: London, 2001).

chapter 3

The why and how of critical appraisal

Julian PL Davis and Iain K Crombie

Introduction

Why should we be critical?

There are many valid reasons for cultivating a healthy scepticism about the results of scientific research. In order to be able to do so consistently and successfully, a sound background knowledge of the design and conduct of research studies is needed. Accepted treatments may be very effective; however, they may also be ineffective or dangerous. If the origin of a treatment has been 'lost in the mists of time', it is often accepted that it has been tried, tested and found to work.

Almost all scientific studies are flawed in some way as it is difficult, if not impossible, to design and conduct a perfect study. For example, a critical assessment of reviews of the appropriateness of prophylactic third molar removal was carried out. The authors identified twelve published reviews, all of which had methodological flaws. The primary studies identified in these reviews were also either flawed, or so poorly reported that it was not possible to draw conclusions from them.[1] The important task is to determine whether those flaws which are inevitably present actually invalidate the findings of the study.

The view from the past

The view that clinical practice should have a basis in research findings is a relatively recent concept. Previous paradigms have included folk beliefs, and the notion that clinical experience is sufficient to guarantee effectiveness of treatment.

Most cultures over the centuries have held beliefs centred on the ability of certain individuals to cure illness. Many early manuscripts contain evidence of treatments and procedures in common use at the time of their writing. Box 3.1 shows a recipe for a dentifrice, quoted in a 1920 text on medieval medicine,[2] originally from a manuscript written by Guy de Chauliac, a French physician practising in around 1350.

This treatment was accepted at the time as a useful and probably effective means of keeping teeth clean and disease-free, and even today, whilst perhaps not the dentists' first choice, would be usable if no altern-ative existed. An intriguing aside is that de Chauliac insists that it is the use of the scarlet cloth which makes the treatment effective. Scarlet was a term used to describe a fine type of cloth, possibly of wool or silk, rather than a reference to its colour. The medieval context was very dif-ferent from our own!

It is not surprising that treatments from as long ago as the 14th century seem unusual to us now. However, as recently as the late 1920s, clinical textbooks still advocated the use of arsenic and dilute hydrochloric acid as a treatment for pellagra, and that newly-popularized triumph of physics, x-rays, as a treatment for asthma.[3] The current view is that there should be some justification in the scientific

Box 3.1 A medieval example

$\frac{1}{2}$ pound sal ammoniac

$\frac{1}{2}$ pound rock salt

$\frac{1}{4}$ pound saccharin alum

crush and dissolve

'The teeth should be rubbed with it, using a little scarlet cloth for the purpose'.

literature for the use of a particular treatment. However, even today, the quality of much of published research is poor, and many current treatments are in fact still based upon received wisdom.

The aim of this chapter is to provide a basic introduction to the interpretation of research studies, and to demystify some aspects of interpreting their findings. It also aims to provide a basic knowledge of how to spot some of the more common faults in published studies. It will assist you in developing a healthy scepticism about 'received wisdom', and 'accepted practice', and make you better able to judge the quality of a piece of research before you accept its conclusions and its relevance to your patients.

Why things go wrong

Studies may produce inaccurate or misleading results because the study methodology is flawed in the design phase, in data collection or in analysis. There will always be instances in which deliberate deception has been practised, in the form of plagiarism or data fabrication. However, the majority of errors are inadvertent, and usually arise from poor design, and a failure to recognize the importance of a number of influential factors. These are as follows.

Chance

The outcome of a research study is subject to the play of chance. The same study repeated under identical conditions (if that were possible) would not necessarily produce the same result.

To illustrate this, let's say we randomly select four samples of 20 people each. The first sample might contain 15 people with dental caries and five without, the second eight with and 12 without, the third 11 with and nine without and the fourth six with and 14 without. These samples vary in their estimates of the prevalence of caries, but overall, we have selected 40 people with caries and 40 without. Combining the samples has provided a more accurate estimate. If enough events are recorded, the effects of chance will be minimized. Studies using small samples may not have sufficient subjects to negate the effects of chance variations.

Bias

A biased sample is one which is systematically non-representative of the population from which it is drawn. One of the more common examples is 'selection bias', in which the sample upon which the research has been carried out may not be representative of the population from which it is drawn. For example, let us assume that a study has shown that recurrence rates of abscess are higher in patients attending a hospital clinic than in those attending their general dental practitioner. The researchers conclude that there is some failing in the hospital treatment which accounts for this. In fact, it is likely that those attending the hospital already have more severe disease, and that they have already been to their dentist and been referred to the hospital clinic.

Confounding

In some cases, the obvious explanation of the results of a study may not be the correct one. The interpretation may miss some underlying factor which accounts for the differences seen, but does not in fact have any involvement in the outcome. Table 3.1 shows some data from a fictitious trial in which the effect of brushing the teeth with a new toothpaste was compared with a placebo, in terms of numbers of fillings needed at the next dental appointment. The sample was divided into those who complied well with the instructions, and those who did not.

Table 3.1 Confounding

	Intervention (fillings per patient)	Placebo (fillings per patient)
Good compliers	0.8	1.0
Poor compliers	3.5	3.7

If you look only at the data from the intervention group, you would conclude that since good compliers have fewer fillings, the treatment must be effective. However, as the study concluded, the same difference is evident in the placebo group, suggesting that there is another factor which is actually influencing both trial groups.

In this case it may be that the sort of people who regularly brush their teeth are also the sort of people who are good at looking after their general health, and do not eat too much sugar or chocolate.

Flawed interpretation

Even if a study has been carefully planned and executed, it is still possible that the authors will draw the wrong conclusions from the data. It may be that they have genuinely overlooked aspects of the results which have important consequences for the interpretation of their findings. It may also be that they have come to the project with a preconceived idea of what they will find, and are – consciously or subconsciously – interpreting the data to suit this view.

Assessing studies – questions to ask

In order to be able to assess whether or not a study is of high quality, there are a number of questions that you should ask. These may be broadly divided into two areas – methodology and interpretation, that is to say those directed at the way the study was designed and conducted, and those aimed at the conclusions drawn from it. There are of course many more questions that could be added to this list, but this gives a basis from which to develop.

Questions of methodology
Aims
Do the authors clearly and unambiguously state the aims of the study? If they do, it becomes easier to assess whether or not they have achieved them. If they do not, the conclusions they draw at the end may be open to criticism, since the question 'Did the study achieve its aims?' cannot

easily be answered. Further, the researchers may be led to report chance (and possibly spurious) findings as if they had been anticipated.

The sample

There are two aspects to this question. Firstly, was the sample size worked out carefully in advance, and was it sufficiently large to allow the statistical conclusions being drawn from it? Secondly, was the sample carefully selected?

The size of a sample is crucial to the ability of a study to achieve its stated aims. As the hypothetical example in Table 3.2 shows, the size of the sample crucially affects the ability of a study to detect small changes in outcome. In general, the larger the sample, the smaller the change that can be picked up. The effects of most treatments are relatively small (for example, a reduction in caries of 10% with a new toothpaste would be looked upon as a huge improvement). This means that most studies need relatively large samples in order to detect reliably changes in outcome.

The key point about selecting a sample is that any conclusions drawn about those selected should be generalizable to the population as a whole. This relies upon the assumption that the composition of sample and population are the same, but often there are systematic differences between the two (bias). There are many ways of selecting a sample of subjects from a population. The scope of this chapter does not allow an exhaustive survey, but a brief mention of some of the more commonly encountered problems will be useful.

Table 3.2

Reduction in numbers of caries at next appointment	Number of subjects needed to detect this reduction
20%	250
10%	1,000
5%	4,000

Using a group of volunteers can be problematic, since those who volunteer are likely to be amongst the most highly motivated individuals, and will provide a highly biased group upon which to test a hypothesis. Likewise, choosing an opportunistic sample, say from patients at one practice, may introduce bias, since the subjects may all share characteristics such as social background. It is important to select an appropriate sampling frame. For example, choosing a sample of patients to test the prevalence of caries from those attending dental practices will overestimate prevalence, since those attending surgeries are likely to be doing so because they have disease. A final point to look out for is the rate of response to the call for subjects. If 5,000 patients were asked to take part, and only 500 actually agreed to do so, those 500 may well be unrepresentative of the population as a whole.

Outcome assessment

The authors of research studies should show that they have made a fair and objective assessment of the outcome of the study. It is all too easy for researchers to fit observations to their preconceived conclusions, rather than the other way round. There are a number of areas in which particular attention should be given to objectivity.

The outcome measure chosen for a study is extremely important. Often, a proxy measure is chosen to represent the actual outcome because the actual outcome is difficult or unethical to assess. It is common to see a study measuring, for example, blood serum levels, when what is really important is the effect on the patient in terms of reduced mortality or improved quality of life. However, it is also important to recognize that just because something is shown to be effective in changing the measured variable in the setting of a trial, or in the laboratory, does not mean that it will be effective in treating patients. Equally, a treatment's ability to alter the proxy measure does not always mean that it will have the desired effect on the health of the patients.

Some attempt should be made to ensure that what is intended to be measured is actually measured. Diagnosis should be supported by some form of comparative test, a 'gold standard', to ensure that the patients being included actually suffer from the condition under study. In addition, measurement of outcome must also be supported by independent expertise, and closely defined before the study is started.

Statistics
Have the statistical methods used been described in detail, and are they the right tests to use in the circumstances? Using the wrong test may indicate spurious significance. Equally, if the authors indicate that they have used a number of more obscure statistical methods, be aware that this may be because the simpler ones didn't produce the results they wanted to show!

Many readers may find that they do not have the requisite statistical expertise to interpret the various tests which are used in research studies. The answer to this is that if you wish to use the findings of a study for use in your own work, and do not feel you have the expertise to decide whether or not the statistical analysis is either appropriate or accurate, show it to a friendly statistician and ask for their advice.

Unforeseen disasters and losses to follow up
If the study ran in to problems, this may result in gaps in the data. Unforeseen events can make it impossible to achieve initial aims.

For example, let us imagine a study looking at the differences in effectiveness of two treatments for gingivitis. The study randomized patients to one of two intervention groups. As the study progressed, it was discovered that a number of patients in the first group found the treatment tasted awful, and stopped taking it. The result was that the first group lost over 40% of its patients to follow up. The researchers can no longer draw reliable conclusions about the comparative effectiveness of the two treatments, only that the remaining treatment was or was not effective in treating gingivitis.

If this sort of thing has happened, the authors should be honest about it in their writing up. In general, however, if something has happened to make the authors change the methodology part way through the study – beware!

In practice, most studies will lose subjects during the course of the work, due to death, migration or loss of interest. These will vary with the population under study. Work on elderly patients will clearly be more likely to suffer from losses due to death and incapacity, especially in longer studies. These losses usually result in bias, since it is often the case that those lost are all similar in some respects. In general, the fewer losses to follow up, the better; but alarm bells should begin to ring if figures above 30% are encountered.

Questions of interpretation

What do the findings mean and what conclusions do the authors draw from them?

People who undertake research studies usually believe strongly in what they are trying to demonstrate. This is beneficial in that it engenders dedication, but it can also be detrimental in that it can make it hard to admit that the results are not what were expected. There may be an important distinction between the actual meaning of the findings, and the spin which the authors may place upon them. You should ask yourself what the findings actually mean. Use the findings, alongside any tables and figures, to draw your own conclusion, and then see what the authors thought the data showed! If there are discrepancies, these may be pointers to problems encountered during the project. It is also at this point that the real reasons for doing the research may show up, with evidence of preconceived ideas, and wishful interpretation.

In some cases, the hoped for conclusion does not materialize. For any number of reasons, the study may show no significant difference between intervention and control groups. In the best traditions of research, this should be met with a fatalistic acceptance, and an attempt to explain why the intervention had no effect. Again, in the worst cases, there may be a rash of tenuous explanations, and attempts to squeeze the weakest but desired conclusion out of unforthcoming data.

One common example of this is 'subgroup analysis'. If the researchers look hard enough, they will find a group of people somewhere in their study whose data show a significant result. Chance will dictate that if you look at enough small subgroups, one of them will turn up a significant result. For example, a trial may have looked at the effect of a novel treatment for caries. The overall result was negative, in that the new treatment was shown to be no better than the old alternative. However, in men between the ages of 25 and 32, the new treatment was better. This type of interpretation is unhelpful, as there was probably another subgroup where the new treatment performed worse, contributing to the overall impression that there was no real difference between treatments.

Another aspect of this is that the researchers may find it hard to bring themselves to accept that the study has categorically shown that their hypothesis was wrong. They may simply ignore the bigger picture and concentrate instead on minutiae, which could be interpreted as supporting their point of view. They may do the opposite, and overlook data which actually supports their conclusions, but does so from a slightly different angle than the one they had hoped for.

Are the results comparable with those found in other literature?
Once you are satisfied that the study has in fact been done carefully, and that the conclusions are likely to be sound, the next step is to compare them with other published studies. If the study in question shows a treatment effect which is much larger than any other trial in the literature, it may be time to be sceptical. It is, of course, possible that the result is true, and that the effect really is larger. Equally, it may be an error of methodology or interpretation.

The findings of a study need to be interpreted in the context of the literature in the field. The references that authors cite are often those which support their point of view. Before accepting the findings, you should also make yourself aware of the results of other studies, and whether or not the current work supports or contradicts them.

Are the findings of any relevance to you in your practice?
The main reason for you as a practising dentist to look at research findings is to decide whether the treatment or intervention under study is of benefit to your patients. Is the overall conclusion that treatment A is better than treatment B of use to you? Is there evidence that this is a real effect? If so, then you should proceed to assess the quality of the study to determine how well the work was done, and the likelihood of the findings being accurate. Lastly, and most importantly, look to see

whether your patients are the same as the subjects of the study (age range, sex ratio, social background), and whether the work was carried out in a similar setting (primary or secondary care, inner city or small town). If not, the findings of the research, however carefully conducted and interpreted, may not be applicable to your patients.

Different study designs need different approaches

Although many of the points covered above are relevant to all study designs, it is useful to highlight some of the more specific areas appropriate to each main type of study.

Surveys

A survey aims to gather data from an identified group, usually by means of a questionnaire or interview, and to use the data to draw conclusions about those people. There are two main questions to be asked:

- is the sample appropriate and carefully chosen to be representative?
- how many people were invited to take part, and how many actually did so?

If the sample is not appropriate (for example asking people with no teeth of their own how they treat toothache) the results will not be generalizable. If there is a poor response rate to the questionnaire (70% plus is good, < 50% is suspect), the chances are good that the sample will be biased, as those who don't reply may be similar in some way.

Cohort studies

A cohort study identifies a group of people of interest, and then follows them through time to observe the natural history of disease. There are two main questions here:

- who is in the sample, and should they be there?
- have the patients been adequately followed up to assess the effects of the study's interventions?

As before, the selection of the sample is vital. In most cohort studies, a control group allows the researchers to assess whether the effects they see in the study group are the result of their interventions, or have occurred as a result of chance events outside the control of the study. If many of the patients have been lost to the follow up process, bias is likely, and the generalizability of the results will be compromised.

Randomized controlled trials

This is the design of choice to assess the effectiveness of new treatments. There are three main questions to be asked:

■ were the subjects randomly allocated to the treatment groups?
■ what were the losses to follow up?
■ were the outcomes of the research assessed blind?

Random allocation helps to ensure that the groups will be evenly balanced at the start of the study. As before, large losses to follow up, especially if they occur particularly in one group, will invalidate conclusions. The need for blinding is especially important as ideally neither those giving nor receiving the treatment should know which group a patient is in, helping to reduce the possible influence of observer bias.

Checklists, and what should be on them

Checklists can make the assessment of research simpler and more repeatable. Using a checklist to assess a number of studies means that the same questions will be asked of each, and the answers will be couched in comparable terms.

Checklists come in a wide variety of forms. They can be very simple, if all the researcher is interested in is, for example, whether the studies were randomized and blinded. At the other end of the scale, they can include many questions on details of the studies, allowing very fine discrimination between them. Checklists will also vary dependent upon the type of study being assessed. As we have indicated above, a list assessing controlled trials needs to include different questions from one assessing cohort studies. If both types are to be included in an appraisal, both sets of questions should be included in the checklist. Boxes 3.2 and 3.3 give a series of possible questions about methodology and interpretation which might form the basis of an assessment checklist.

Box 3.2 Methodology

Aims and design
Was there a clearly stated aim for the research?
Was the study design appropriate for the task?
Was the study designed properly?

Sample
Was the sample carefully selected?
Did the sample represent the population in question?
Was the sample size properly calculated?

Uncontrollable influences
Did the researchers consider the effects of bias, chance and confounding on their results?
Did any patients receive other treatments, or suffer other ailments?

Control group
Should there be a control group?
Was there a control group?
Was it appropriately selected?

Randomization and blinding
Were subjects randomly allocated?
Was the randomization carefully conducted?
Was randomization blinded?
Was treatment blinded/double blinded?

Measurements and statistical tests
Were the things being measured clinically relevant?
Were they measured accurately and consistently?
Was there a 'gold standard' for diagnosis or measurement?
Were details given of statistical tests used?
Were these appropriate?
Was the statistical analysis carried out blind to intervention?

Completeness of the study and unforeseen problems
Were losses to follow up acceptable?
Were attempts made to retrieve lost subjects?
How complete was the data set?
Had the methodology changed during the study in response to unforeseen circumstances?
Have the researchers admitted problems and tried to tackle them?

Box 3.3 Interpretation

Findings
What were the findings of the study?
Has the study achieved its aim?
What do the authors conclude?

Interpretation
Do the researchers interpret the findings correctly?
Have they attempted to cover up shortfalls in the data?
Do they draw untenable conclusions?

Errors of interpretation
Has important data been ignored/overlooked?
Has unreliable data been included?

Generalizability
Are the conclusions applicable to a wider patient group?
Is the conclusion relevant to my patients?

Summary

Cultivating a critical attitude to research studies is an essential skill in interpreting the current flood of publications. As the evidence based dentistry movement develops and becomes an integral part of everyday practice, it will become central to successful dentistry that every practitioner can read and assess published studies. There is no need for each dentist to be an expert in appraisal of research, but an awareness of the basics, and an idea of which questions to ask, will be invaluable.

References

1. Song F, Landes DP, Glenny A-M, Sheldon TA, Prophylactic removal of impacted third molars: an assessment of published reviews, *Br Dent J* (1997) **182**:339–346.

2. Walsh JJ, *Mediaeval Medicine* (A & C Black: London, 1920).
3. Beeson PB, Changes in medical therapy during the past half century, *Medicine* (1980) **59**:79–99.

Further reading

This chapter is intended to be a brief introduction to critical appraisal. If you wish to pursue this in more depth, the following sources are a good place to start.

Crombie IK, *A Pocket Guide to Critical Appraisal* (BMJ Publishing Group: London, 1996).
Greenhalgh T, *How to Read a Paper* (BMJ Publishing Group: London,1997).
Greenhalgh T, Donald A, *Evidence-Based Heatlhcare Workbook: Understanding Research* (BMJ Publishing Group: London, 2000).
Li Wan Po A, *Dictionary of Evidence-Based Medicine* (Radcliffe Medical Press: Oxford, 1998).
Locke LF, Silverman SJ, Spirduso WW, *Reading and Understanding Research* (Sage Publications: London,1998).
Sackett DL, Richardson WS, Rosenberg, W, *Evidence-Based Medicine – How to Practice and Teach EBM* (Churchill Livingstone: London, 1997).
Streiner DL, Norman GR, *PDQ Epidemiology* (Mosby: St Louis, 1996).

chapter 4

Why are systematic reviews useful?

Anne-Marie Glenny and Lee Hooper

As the importance of evidence based practice continues to be promoted, so the profile of the systematic review prospers. The process of conducting a systematic review involves 'locating, appraising, and synthesizing evidence from scientific studies in order to provide informative empirical answers to scientific research questions'.[1] In the late 1980s, Mulrow highlighted that many traditional medical reviews were haphazard and biased, often reflecting the opinion of the review's authors.[2] In contrast, systematic reviews follow explicit, well documented, scientific methodology in order to reduce both systematic errors (biases) and random errors (those occurring by chance), and to provide a more objective, comprehensive view of the research literature.

Why are systematic reviews important? The rationale for systematic reviews has been well documented.[3,4] In addition to the reduction in bias, one of the many advantages of systematic reviews is that they enable us to reduce the ever-increasing torrent of both published and unpublished research literature into manageable portions. In dentistry alone there are around 500 journals publishing over 43,000 research articles a year. It is unfeasible to expect anyone to keep abreast of the emerging research evidence, identifying those articles that are both of a high quality and relevant to their own clinical practice.

Systematic reviews can be used to formulate policy and develop guidelines on the organization and delivery of health care. They are of particular benefit in areas of clinical uncertainty or where there is a wide variation in practice. Healthcare providers, researchers and policy makers can use systematic reviews to efficiently integrate existing information, providing data for rational decision making.

Systematic reviews can be used not only to inform clinical decision making, but also to inform the research agenda. The comprehensive searching, appraising and synthesizing of research literature does not guarantee a definitive answer to a scientific research question. By identifying questions for which, at present, there is insufficient good-quality evidence upon which to base clinical decisions, systematic reviews can highlight areas requiring further primary research. Conversely, the results of systematic review may provide strong evidence regarding the benefits or harms of a particular intervention and may actually preclude a new study from being conducted. Funding bodies are increasingly demanding that applicants proposing new trials justify the need for such trials in light of relevant systematic reviews.

A systematic review may, or may not, contain a meta-analysis. Meta-analysis refers to statistical analysis of the results from independent studies. Such analysis usually aims to produce a single estimate of treatment effect. The quantitative pooling of data from individual studies leads to an increase in sample size and an increase in power, which is particularly important when the size of effect is small or there is a relatively low event rate.[3] The increase in sample size not only means an increase in power, but also an increase in the precision in the estimate of effect, demonstrated by the narrowing of associated confidence intervals. Meta-analysis should only be conducted where appropriate, for example where significant heterogeneity between studies does not exist. If significant heterogeneity is shown to exist, differences in study characteristics (for example, differences in the participants, interventions or settings included in the primary studies) should be explored qualitatively. Meta-analysis will be explored further in Chapter 5.

In recent years, the interest in systematic reviews, their production and publication has been growing. Yet, despite the well documented advantages of this scientific technique, some are still doubtful about the usefulness of such reviews. These doubts are often based upon misconceptions regarding the 'history, purpose, methods and uses of systematic reviews'.[5] Common misconceptions are that systematic reviews include only randomized, controlled trials; that they can be done without experienced information/library support; that they necessarily involve statistical synthesis; and that they are only interested in disease outcomes.

In order to further promote the role of systematic reviews and dispel the criticism aimed at them, it is imperative that those undertaking systematic reviews ensure that the reviews are robust, and follow a rigorous, 'transparent' protocol.

Where will I find systematic reviews?

Systematic reviews are published in many medical and dental journals, and indexed by a variety of electronic databases, such as MEDLINE and EMBASE. The problem is that with so many other articles of different types (trials, case studies, ordinary reviews, letters, etc.), it is difficult to find systematic reviews, either by browsing through journals or by searching on MEDLINE.

The best solution is to search the Cochrane Library, which contains two databases dedicated to helping you locate the systematic review you need. The Cochrane Database of Systematic Reviews (CDSR) includes full-text systematic reviews that have been completed to the exacting standards of the Cochrane Collaboration, and protocols of reviews that are under way. The Database of Abstracts of Reviews of Effectiveness (DARE) is produced by the NHS Centre for Reviews and Dissemination (CRD), and is a compilation of abstracts of systematic reviews that are published in paper journals, along with helpful commentary on their quality.

One search on the Cochrane Library *(see Chapter 2 on searching)* allows you to scan through the systematic reviews held on both of these databases, without having to wade through all the other studies in your subject area.

So what does a systematic review consist of?

This section describes the stages that a reviewer has moved through to produce a systematic review, and is illustrated with examples from a completed systematic review.[6] Once you have found a systematic review in your subject, this section (and Chapter 5 on meta-analysis) will help you to understand and evaluate it. However, if you intend to conduct or commission a review then you require much more detail, and will need to also read one or both of the essential manuals, the *Cochrane Reviewer's Handbook*[7] or CRD Report number 4.[1] Also, if you are producing a systematic review to be published in a peer-reviewed journal, you may be asked to adhere to the QUOROM statement guidelines.[8]

The use of a **tightly defined set of explicit systematic methods** in reviewing helps to minimize the biases (systematic errors) and random errors that can otherwise creep into reviews. The following are the steps that should have been followed.

The first step in a systematic review is to specify a clearly focused **question**. For example, a question on the effectiveness of an intervention would be phrased in terms of:

- population (group to whom the intervention will apply),
- intervention (the therapy, treatment or preventive policy to be carried out),
- comparison (what will the intervention be compared against? – it could be a common alternative intervention, a placebo or no intervention), and
- outcomes (what do we wish to measure at the end, what is important to us and to consumers?).

An example of a focused question for a systematic review is shown in Box 4.0. This question is stated upfront and explicitly, allowing you, the potential user of the review, to decide quickly whether it addresses **your** question – will the review be useful to you?

The process of creating a systematic review should begin with a clear **protocol** describing the background to the work, the hypothesis to be tested and the methodology to be used – just like any other scientific

Box 4.0 Focused question and inclusion criteria for a systematic review – an example[6]

To assess the effectiveness of interventions (which may include placebo or no treatment) for the treatment of oral mucositis, or its associated pain, for patients with cancer receiving chemotherapy and/or radiotherapy

The question should be used to develop criteria by which studies will be assessed for their relevance to the review. The type of study design(s) to be included in the review should also be stated.

Population
Anyone with cancer who is receiving chemotherapy and/or radiotherapy and has oral mucositis

Intervention
Any active intervention for the treatment of oral mucositis or its associated pain

Comparison
Placebo, no treatment or another active intervention

Outcomes
Mucositis at different levels of severity
Oral pain scores or categories
Relief of dysphagia
Incidence of systemic infection
Amount of analgesia
Stay in hospital (days)
Cost of oral care
Patient quality of life

Study design
Only randomized, controlled trials were eligible for the review

study. The protocol limits bias by allowing peer (and often consumer) review of the question to be asked and methods to be used. This helps to prevent studies with 'good' results being preferentially included, or data dredging (where lots of analyses are tried out, but only those with significant results reported) being practised. Once the systematic review has been published you will no longer have access to the protocol, but the review itself may refer to the protocol and a clear, logical line of progress should be discernible.

Ideally **inclusion and exclusion criteria** are specified in the protocol and then reflected later in the completed review. These criteria should relate closely to the question asked (Box 4.0). Besides the population, intervention, comparison and outcomes that should be represented in the inclusion and exclusion criteria, the type of studies will be specified. Ideally, these will be the studies that offer the least-biased evidence for the review. For questions of therapy, this is usually the randomized, controlled trial, but other types of study are better suited to answer different questions. Ideally, the process of deciding on inclusion of studies is performed independently by at least two people, on a form specifically designed for the review.

If a systematic review is to represent a good summary of current evidence on the chosen question, then it must use a transparent and inclusive **search strategy**, aiming to include all the published, and preferably also unpublished, data that exist (Box 4.1). Ideally, several types of search are adopted, so that, if one strategy misses a relevant study, it may be picked up through another searching method. Search strategies generally include several of the following: structured searches of several electronic databases (including the Cochrane Library), checks through the reference lists of included studies and relevant reviews, letters to relevant pharmaceutical companies and experts in the field asking about unpublished or ongoing work, hand searching of relevant journals or conference abstracts, and translation of foreign-language articles.

There is good evidence of publication bias according to the results of a study – those with statistically significant results are more likely to be submitted for publication,[9,10] more likely to be published in English-language journals,[11] and more likely to be published sooner[12] than studies with more equivocal results. So, if only the most easily accessible studies are included, then the effects of the treatment may be overestimated, as the trials showing less dramatic effects have been left out. For this reason, it is useful to assess whether the authors have checked for bias in the set

Box 4.1 Search strategy for the identification of studies – an example[6]

The search attempted to identify all relevant trials, irrespective of language. Papers not in English were considered and translations carried out by members of the Cochrane Collaboration.

Electronic searching – the databases searched were:
Cochrane Oral Health Group Specialised Register
Cochrane Controlled Trials Register (2001, issue 3)
MEDLINE (from 1966)
EMBASE (from 1974)
Sensitive search strategies were developed for each database (available from the authors, on request) using a combination of free text and MeSH terms.

The search strategy for CCTR is given as an example below:
1. NEOPLASMS*:ME
2. NEOPLASM*
3. CANCER*
4. (TUMOUR* or TUMOR*)
5. MALIGNAN*
6. RADIOTHERAPY*:ME
7. RADIOTH*
8. BONE-MARROW-TRANSPLANTATION:ME
9. ((BONE next MARROW) near TRANSPLANT*)
10. CHEMO*
11. (((((((((#1 or #2) or #3) or #4) or #5) or #6) or #7) or #8) or #9) or #10)
12. STOMATITIS*:ME
13. STOMATITIS
14. CANDIDIASIS-ORAL:ME
15. (ORAL and CAND*)
16. (ORAL and MUCOS*)
17. (ORAL and FUNG*)
18. (((((#12 or #13) or #14) or #15) or #16) or #17)
19. (#11 and #18)

Only hand searching carried out by the Cochrane Collaboration is included in the search (see master list, www.cochrane.org).

The reference list of related review articles and all articles obtained were checked for further trials. Authors of trial reports and specialists in the field known to the reviewers were written to concerning further published and unpublished trials. The review will be updated every two years using CCTR, Cochrane Oral Health Group Specialised Register, MEDLINE, EMBASE and LILACS.

Date of most recent searches: May 2001 (CCTR 2001, issue 2)

of included trials (even after comprehensive searching) by drawing up a funnel plot.

Studies of varying **quality** are performed and published. It is often the case that studies of lower validity suggest more favourable results than those of higher validity.[13] Potential types of bias relating to validity include:

- selection bias (where the process of randomization is subverted so that there are non-random differences between the people allocated to the different experimental groups),
- attrition bias (where more participants drop out of one experimental arm for some reason),
- performance bias (where those receiving the intervention and/or those caring for them are aware of the experimental allocation and may alter concurrent treatments accordingly), and
- detection bias (where those assessing outcomes are aware of the experimental allocation and may be open to biased outcome measurement).[7]

Assessment of study validity (preferably independently duplicated) and some statement on how those biases may affect outcomes are essential in understanding the believability of the results of a systematic review, so look out for how quality was assessed when you read a systematic review (Box 4.2). Sensitivity analyses (leaving out certain studies when pooling data to discover if this radically alters the results of the review), in which low-quality studies are dropped from the analysis, can be helpful in understanding how robust the results of the review really are. It is important that the results of the review reflect the results of the included studies, and also an element of the quality of the studies. If the quality of included studies is low, then the quality of the 'answer' can be no better.

Extracting data from studies may sometimes involve arbitrary decisions and mistakes that can result in random error or bias. Where data extraction is independently duplicated, and the criteria for making the decisions pre-specified (in the protocol), we can be more confident that bias is not creeping into the review. Data extraction should also be comprehensive (on a

Box 4.2 Quality assessment – an example[6]

The quality assessment of included trials was undertaken independently and in duplicate by two reviewers as part of the data-abstraction process. Included trials were assessed on three criteria: concealed allocation of treatment (A = adequate, B = unclear, C = inadequate), blinding of patients, providers and outcome assessors, and information on reasons for withdrawal by intervention group.

The concealment of allocation was adequate for only three (20%) of the 15 trials and it was unclear for the remaining 12. In five trials assessing pain, the patient could not be blinded to the intervention. The outcome assessor was blind for the remaining 10 trials. Nine trials gave a clear description of withdrawals by trial group, this being unclear in the remaining trials.

There is weak and unreliable evidence that allopurinol mouthwash and vitamin E may be beneficial in curing mucositis.

Box 4.3 Data extraction – an example[6]

Data were extracted by two reviewers independently, using specially designed data-extraction forms. The characteristics of the trial participants, interventions and outcomes in the included trials are presented in the study tables. Mucositis may be dichotomized at different levels of severity. In order to maximize the availability of similar outcome data, we recorded the number of patients in each category of mucositis. Pain was assessed on visual analogue scales (0 to 100), and the means and standard deviations for each group were recorded. The duration of trials and timing of assessments were recorded in order to make a decision about which to include for commonality. We also recorded the country in which the trial was conducted and whether a dentist was involved in the investigation. Authors were contacted for clarification or for further information.

form designed for the review) and clearly tabulated to allow transparency and possibly corrections at a later date. Ideally, the reviewers will have contacted the study authors to fill in any gaps in published reports, so that best possible use is made of the data that exist (Box 4.3).

Pooling of data is usually narrative, and may also involve statistical pooling or meta-analysis (see the next chapter). The decision to stay with a narrative data pooling or add in a meta-analysis is generally made by referring to guidelines set down in the protocol, and based on a decision as to whether the trials to be pooled appear similar enough for this to be sensible. The review is not necessarily of higher quality because it contains a meta-analysis. In many cases it is better not to meta-analyse. Narrative or meta-analytic comparisons and sub-groupings should have been pre-specified in the protocol (to avoid multiple analyses being carried out with only the 'statistically significant' ones being published). An example of the presentation of both narrative and statistical pooling of results is presented in Box 4.4.

Meta-analysis aims to pool extracted numerical data, weighted so that larger studies, or those with less variability, contribute more to the outcome. This pooling provides an answer with greater precision than each included study on its own. The meta-analysis itself may use fixed-effects (where it is assumed that the true outcomes of the various studies are the same) or random-effects methodologies (where the true outcomes are assumed to vary a little with differing study inclusion, dose, duration, etc.). Heterogeneity of studies (differences in study characteristics and/or large differences in results) is ideally explored through sub-grouping or meta-regression. This allows those characteristics of studies that alter the results to be discerned – for example, a treatment may work better in older adults and poorly in young adults. This type of information is especially helpful, as it can allow practitioners to fit treatment decisions to individuals in their care.

Box 4.4 Pooling of data – an example[6]

Four placebo-controlled trials, using three active agents (allopurinol mouthwash, tetrachlorodecaoxide, benzydamine mouthwash), reported effectiveness, as improvement or not, of mucositis. Only one trial (n = 44) reported a significant improvement in mucositis for the test compared with the control group, with allopurinol mouthwash as the active agent, RR = 0.63 (95% CI 0.42 to 0.96). There was no evidence that tetrachlorodecaoxide or benzydamine mouthwash was effective, compared with placebo, at improving mucositis.

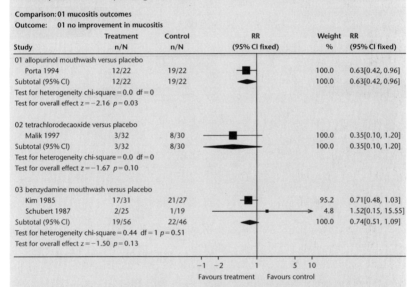

The significance of discrepancies in the estimates of the treatment effects from the different trials was assessed by means of Cochran's test for heterogeneity. If any significant heterogeneity ($p < 0.1$) was detected, it was planned to re-assess the significance of the treatment effects by using a random-effects model; however, no heterogeneity was found.

Results of the review should ideally be clearly presented, often tabulated (Table 4.1), along with details of the primary studies, an assessment of validity and results of sensitivity analyses. The results should be reflected directly in the conclusions drawn.

Table 4.1 Table of characteristics of included studies – an example[6]

Study ID	Coda 1997	Dodd 2000
Methods	Randomized, double-blind. Eligible patients had oral mucositis and had been on opioids for at least 2 days. Clear information given on withdrawals.	Randomized, double-blind. Patient had mucositis confirmed by clinician. Unclear information on withdrawals.
Participants	Adults with mixed cancer having BMT, including TBI. 119 enrolled, 97 completed.	Adults with mixed cancer treated with stomatotoxic chemotherapy excluding radiation treatment, leukaemia or BMT. 299 eligible, 200 enrolled, 142 completed.
Interventions	Three groups, all using patient-controlled analgesia (PCA). Groups: Morphine 5 mg/ml; Hydromorphone 1 mg/ml; Sufentanil 5 μg/ml for up to 20 days.	Three mouthwash groups, all with oral training programme. Soda and salt, 1 tsp/pint. Chlorhexidine 0.12%. Magic-lidocaine 0.5%, diphenhydramine HCL 0.25 ml. Aluminium hydroxide 14.75 ml. 20 ml swish 20 s 4 times/day.
Outcomes	Average pain VAS score (0–100) for days 2–5. Number who discontinued as drug not working. Other outcomes.	Patient soreness rating on VAS score (0–10) for 7 days, day 7 used. Mucositis oral assessment guide used by patients dichotomized as eradicated or not.
Notes		Converted VAS scale to 0–100.
Allocation concealment	Adequate.	Unclear.

How can I tell if this is a good systematic review?

Unfortunately, not all published systematic reviews are of a high quality (with quality being defined as the confidence that the design, conduct and analysis of the review minimized biases).[1] It is important, therefore, to undertake critical appraisal of any systematic review before acting on its findings. The main issues regarding the quality of a review are closely linked to the steps involved in the review process, outlined above. A list of the key issues to be examined when appraising a review article are outlined in Box 4.5.

Box 4.5 Critically appraising review articles

1. **What are the review's objectives?**
   A good review should focus on well defined questions, stating the populations, intervention/control groups, and outcomes to be included.
2. **How comprehensive was the search strategy?**
   The reviewers should make a substantial effort to search for all the literature relevant to the question. Published and unpublished literature should be searched for; any restrictions regarding language of publication should be stated and justified, as should the time period covered by the search. Ideally, a systematic review needs to be up to date, incorporating all the recent literature.
3. **What were the inclusion/exclusion criteria?**
   The criteria for selecting or rejecting studies should be clearly stated and appropriate. The process* by which articles are assessed for relevance should also be recorded.
4. **How was the validity of the primary studies assessed?**
   The process* by which validity assessment was undertaken and the criteria used to assess the quality of the primary studies should be clear. It should also be apparent how the results of the validity assessment are used within the review's data synthesis.
5. **How were data extracted from the primary studies?**
   The process* by which data was extracted from the primary studies should be transparent.

Continued

Box 4.5 *continued*

6. **Are the characteristics of the included studies clearly displayed?**
   A table illustrating the study characteristics of each included primary study should be presented. This allows the reader to view more closely the populations, interventions, mode of delivery, outcomes, settings, etc. that have been examined in the individual studies.
7. **Does the review examine differences/similarities between the included studies and their results?**
   Heterogeneity between studies should be explored and the reasons for any variations discussed. Heterogeneity can be explored statistically, graphically, or through a narrative.
8. **Was the synthesis of the data carried out appropriately?**
   Were data pooled qualitatively or statistically? If statistical pooling (meta-analysis) was used, was it used appropriately? If there is no discussion of heterogeneity within the review, or significant heterogeneity between studies was identified, then the appropriateness of statistical pooling must be examined.
9. **Were the results interpreted appropriately?**
   Any conclusions, implications for research or practice should follow on logically from the results.

*Ideally the assessment of relevance and validity, and data extraction should be carried out independently by two (or more) reviewers and a comment made on how discrepancies were resolved.

Checklists have been published to guide the reader through the process of critically appraising review articles, helping to draw conclusions on the review's validity and generalizability to the local population.[14,15] Only when the quality of the review and its generalizability have been considered should a judgement about the applicability of the review's findings be made.

Further reading

Oxman AD, Cook DJ, Guyatt GH, Users' guides to the medical literature.

II. How to use an overview, *JAMA* (1994) **272**:1367–1371. (Text also available at: http://www.cche.net/userguides/overview.asp)

Critical Appraisal Skills Programme (CASP) website, http://www.phru.org.uk/~casp/index.htm.
(CASP is a UK project that aims to help service decision makers develop skills in the critical appraisal of evidence about effectiveness, in order to promote the delivery of evidence based healthcare).

References

1. NHS Centre for Reviews and Dissemination, *Undertaking Systematic Reviews of Research on Effectiveness: CRD's Guidance for Carrying Out or Commissioning Reviews*, 2nd edn (NHS Centre for Reviews and Dissemination, University of York, 2001).
   Also available at http://www.york.ac.uk/inst/crd.
2. Mulrow CD, The medical review article: state of the science, *Ann Intern Med* (1987) **106**:485–488.
3. Mulrow CD, Rationale for systematic reviews, *BMJ* (1994) **309**:597–599.
4. Chalmers I, Altman D, *Systematic Reviews* (BMJ Publishing Group: London, 1995).
5. Petticrew M. Systematic reviews from astronomy to zoology: myths and misconceptions, *BMJ* (2001) **322**:98–101.
6. Worthington HV, Clarkson JE, Eden OB, Interventions for treating oral mucositis for patients with cancer receiving treatment (Cochrane Review). In: *The Cochrane Library* (Issue 1, Update Software: Oxford, 2002).
7. Clarke M, Oxman A, eds, Cochrane Reviewers' Handbook 4.1 [updated June 2000]. In: *Review Manager (RevMan) – Version 4.1* [Computer program] (The Cochrane Collaboration: Oxford, England, 2000).
   Also available at http://www.cochrane.org/cochrane/hbook.htm.
8. Moher D, Cook D, Eastwood S et al, Improving the quality of reports of meta-analyses of randomised controlled trials: the QUOROM statement, *Lancet* (1999) **354**:1896–1899.
9. Ioannidis J, Effect of the statistical significance of results on the time to completion and publication of randomized efficacy trials, *JAMA* (1998) **279**:281–286.
10. Scherer R, Dickersin K, Langenberg P, Full publication of results initially presented in abstracts: a meta-analysis, *JAMA* (1994) **272**:158–162.
11. Egger M, Zellweger-Zahner T, Schneider M et al, Language bias in randomised controlled trials published in English and German, *Lancet* (1997) **350**:158–162.
12. Stern J, Simes R, Publication bias: evidence of delayed publication in a cohort study of clinical research projects, *BMJ* (1997) **315**:640–645.

13. Linde K, Scholz M, Ramirez A et al, Impact of study quality on outcome in placebo-controlled trials of homeopathy, *J Clin Epidemiol* (1999) **52**:631–636.
14. CASP *Evidence Based Healthcare Workbook (with CD-ROM)* (Updated Software for the Critical Appraisal Skills Programme: Oxford, 1999).
15. Crombie I, *The Pocket Guide to Critical Appraisal: A Handbook for Health Care Professionals* (BMJ Publishing Group: London, 1996).

chapter 5

Understanding the statistical pooling of data

Helen Worthington

Meta-analysis

The pooling of data is frequently known as conducting a meta-analysis of the data. The term 'meta-analysis' was first used in 1976 by Glass to distinguish between the primary analysis of a research study from a secondary re-analysis of the data to answer new research questions.[1] The formal definition in *A Dictionary of Epidemiology* is 'the process of using statistical methods to combine the results of different studies'.[2] Sometimes the term is used to describe the whole process of systematic reviewing. However, in this chapter the definition above will be used where a meta-analysis is confined to the pooling of the data from different studies, usually in a systematic review.

Before conducting a meta-analysis, it is important that the reviewer feels that it is appropriate to pool these studies. It is important that the studies are reasonably similar with respect to such factors as the study patients, the types of intervention and what the intervention is being compared to, and that the outcome measurements are similar, and measured on a similar measurement scale.

The statistical methods for pooling data are fairly straightforward. Statistical techniques have been developed for data measurement on either a binary (dichotomous) or a continuous (interval) scale. Data measured on a binary scale takes only two categories, for example, present or absent, dead or alive, carious or sound. Data measured on a continuous measurement scale takes all possible values along a continuum, where a change of one unit along the scale means the same thing at all points along the scale. Examples of data measured on a continuous scale are: blood pressure, height, weight and loss of attachment (mm). Frequently the measurement scale of the data will be between these two extremes and is ordinal in type i.e. where there is a natural ordering to the measurements, but a change of one unit along the scale does not necessarily mean the same thing at different points along the scale. Examples of data measured on an ordinal scale would be the rating of the success of a dental procedure on a 5-point scale, from failure to complete success. When confronted with data measured on an ordinal scale, the researcher has to decide whether to dichotomize the data, or to treat the data as continuous, before conducting a meta-analysis.

Meta-analysis is used to make relative comparisons between two study groups, one of which is the intervention. This may be compared to a placebo intervention, a no treatment intervention or another intervention. The following two sections describe the estimates of treatment effect used to compare binary and continuous outcomes in individual studies.

Binary data

For binary data the common estimates of treatment effect used to compare the two study groups are the odds ratio (OR) and relative risk (RR) (synonymous with risk ratio), which are relative effects, and risk difference (RD), which is an absolute effect. The formulas for calculating these estimates are given in Table 5.1 and the definitions below are those given in the glossary of the Cochrane Library (Cochrane Library, Issue 1, 2001).

The odds ratio (OR) is the ratio of the odds of an event in the experimental (intervention) group to the odds of an event in the control group. Odds are the ratio of the number of people in a group with an event to the number without an event. Thus, if a group of 100 people had an event rate of 0.20, 20 people had the event and 80 did not, and

Table 5.1 Effect measures for binary data

	Outcome	
	Yes	*No*
Intervention	a	b
Control	c	d

Odds ratio = (a/b)/(c/d)
Relative risk (or risk ratio) (RR) = [a/(a+b)]/[c/(c+d)]
Relative risk reduction = 1 – RR
Risk difference (or absolute risk reduction, ARR) (RD) = a/(a+b) – c/(c+d)
Number needed to treat (NNT) = 1/RD

the odds would be 20/80 or 0.25. An OR of 1 indicates no difference between comparison groups. For undesirable outcomes, an OR that is less than 1 indicates that the intervention was effective in reducing the risk of that outcome. When the event rate is small, odds ratios are very similar to relative risks (Cochrane Library, Issue 1, 2001).

The relative risk (RR) is the ratio of the risk in the intervention group to the risk in the control group. The risk (proportion, probability or rate) is the ratio of people with an event in a group to the total in the group. As with the OR, an RR of 1 indicates no difference between comparison groups, and for undesirable outcomes, an RR that is less than 1 indicates that the intervention was effective in reducing the risk of that outcome.

Odds ratios are preferred by statisticians as they have appealing mathematical properties. However, they are frequently misinterpreted as RR values, which will overestimate the benefit or harm of a treatment. Relative risks are much easier to explain and use and, if everything else is equal, they may be a better measure for clinicians and patients.

The risk difference (RD) is the absolute difference in the event rate between two comparison groups. A risk difference of zero indicates no difference between comparison groups. An RD that is less than zero indicates that the intervention was effective in reducing the risk of that outcome.

Another measure of effect that is sometimes calculated once the study results have been pooled is the number needed to treat (NNT). This uses a summary statistic and it is the number of patients who need to be treated to prevent one bad outcome; it is the inverse of the risk difference. There are problems in using this measure as it is dependent on the baseline risk and, therefore, is sensitive to factors that may change this risk.[3]

Forest plot

In order to begin to combine the result of studies for a binary outcome, it is necessary to have for each study one of these measures of effect, along with its 95% confidence interval. A forest plot consists of this information plotted for each study. The example in Figure 5.1 has been taken from an Oral Health Group review on the Cochrane Library.[4] This review looks at the relative efficacy of anti-fungal agents, compared with either a placebo or no treatment, in the prevention of oral candidiasis in patients with cancer, undergoing chemotherapy. Six studies were included in this meta-analysis, and the relative risk and the 95% confidence interval are shown for each study. In the first study shown in Figure 5.1, Bodey 1990,[5] one patient out of 58 in the anti-fungal drug group acquired oral candidiasis during the chemotherapy treatment compared to 15 out of 54 patients in the placebo group. The relative risk for this study was 0.06, with a 95% confidence interval (0.01, 0.45). In this study, the RR of 0.06 is interpreted as follows: treatment with the anti-fungal drug decreases the number of patients acquiring oral candidiasis by 94% when compared with the control group. It can be seen that wide confidence intervals are associated with smaller studies and larger studies, such as Palmblad 1992,[9] have narrower confidence intervals. At the bottom of the plot, the diamond indicates the summary relative risk of 0.36 along with its 95% confidence interval (0.24, 0.54). The meta-analysis shows that the anti-fungal drugs reduce the number of patients acquiring oral candidiasis by 64% when compared with the control. The weight given to each study in the meta-analysis summary

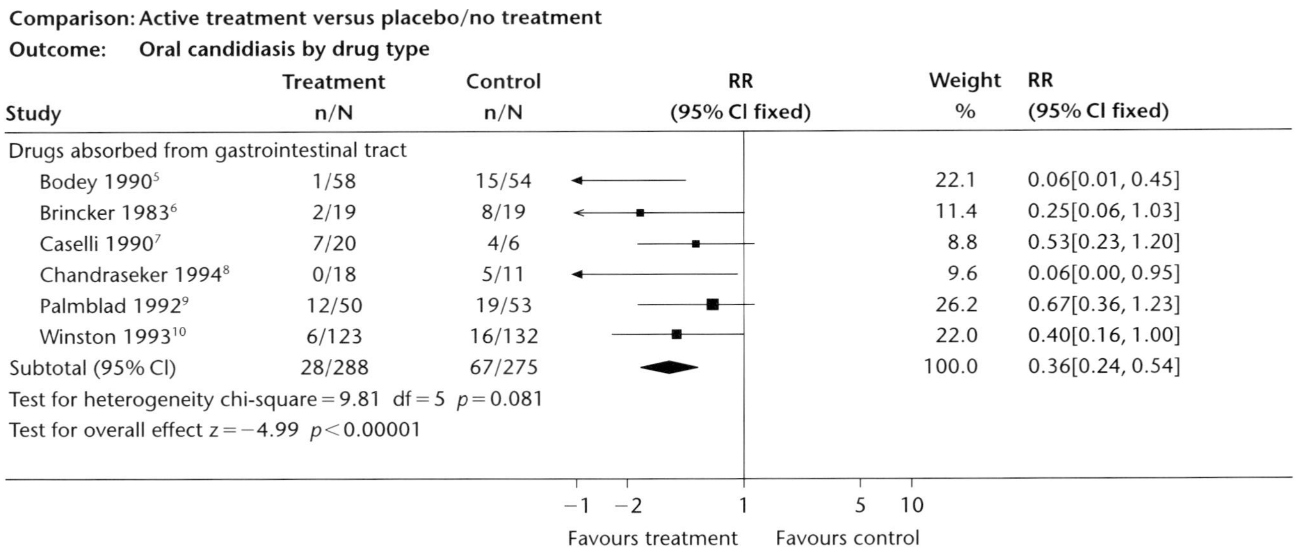

Comparison: Active treatment versus placebo/no treatment

Outcome: Oral candidiasis by drug type

Study	Treatment n/N	Control n/N	RR (95% CI fixed)	Weight %	RR (95% CI fixed)
Drugs absorbed from gastrointestinal tract					
Bodey 1990[5]	1/58	15/54		22.1	0.06[0.01, 0.45]
Brincker 1983[6]	2/19	8/19		11.4	0.25[0.06, 1.03]
Caselli 1990[7]	7/20	4/6		8.8	0.53[0.23, 1.20]
Chandraseker 1994[8]	0/18	5/11		9.6	0.06[0.00, 0.95]
Palmblad 1992[9]	12/50	19/53		26.2	0.67[0.36, 1.23]
Winston 1993[10]	6/123	16/132		22.0	0.40[0.16, 1.00]
Subtotal (95% CI)	28/288	67/275		100.0	0.36[0.24, 0.54]

Test for heterogeneity chi-square = 9.81 df = 5 p = 0.081

Test for overall effect z = −4.99 p < 0.00001

−1   −2   1   5   10

Favours treatment   Favours control

Figure 5.1 *Example of a forest plot for the binary outcome, absence or presence of oral candidiasis, from a review looking at preventing oral candidiasis in patients with cancer undergoing chemotherapy.*[4]

statistics is shown, and this is related to the inverse variance of each relative risk estimate. At the bottom of the forest plot is the p value associated with the overall effect (measured by the z test). In this example $p < 0.00001$, which indicates significance.

Continuous data

For each study, the difference between the study means is calculated, along with the 95% confidence intervals for the mean difference. These studies are then combined so that the weight given to each study (i.e. how much influence each study has on the overall results of the meta-analysis) is determined by the precision of its estimate of effect, and this is frequently equal to the inverse of the variance. Figure 5.2 shows the forest plot for four studies included in a Cochrane Oral Health Group review. This looks at the relative efficacy of guided tissue regeneration (GTR) compared with conventional open flap surgery, in relation to attachment level change (mm) over 12 months.[11] The review pools data from four parallel groups and six split-mouth studies. However, to simplify the presentation of the data, the data for the parallel group studies only are shown here. Once again the raw study data for each group are shown to the left of the plot, enabling readers to examine it. The diamond at the bottom summarizes the pooled weighted mean difference (WMD) across the studies, with the horizontal length of the diamond indicating the 95% confidence interval. In this example the weighted mean difference is 1.52 (95% CI: 1.16, 1.88).

Heterogeneity

As previously discussed, the reviewer must feel confident about combining the studies to be included in a meta-analysis. Once this has been done, it is extremely important to assess whether the studies can be considered to be similar or not. Heterogeneous studies will be spread out, with the 95% confidence intervals for each study not overlapping with

Comparison: GTR

Outcome: Attachment level change

Study	Treatment n	Treatment mean(SD)	Control n	Control mean(SC)	WMD (95%CI fixed)	Weight %	WMD (95%CI fixed)
Cortellini 1995[12]	30	4.70(2.10)	15	2.50(0.80)		17.9	2.20[1.35, 3.05]
Cortellini 1996[13]	24	4.90(1.30)	12	2.30(0.80)		27.4	2.60[1.91, 3.29]
Mayfield 1998[14]	20	1.30(2.10)	18	1.10(1.80)		8.5	0.20[−1.04, 1.44]
Tonetti 1998[15]	69	3.04(1.64)	64	2.18(1.48)		46.3	0.86[0.33, 1.39]
Total (95%CI)	143		109			100.0	1.52[1.16,1.88]

Test for heterogeneity chi-square = 22.16 df = 3 p = 0.0001

Test for overall effect z = 8.26 p < 0.00001

−4   −2   0   2   4

Favours treatment   Favours control

Figure 5.2 *Example of meta-analysis for the continuous outcome, change in level of attachment, for four parallel group studies from a review comparing guided tissue regeneration (GTR) with conventional open flap surgery.*[11]

other studies. In Figure 5.2, the four studies included in the guided tissue regeneration review appear to be heterogeneous.[12-15] The formal chi-square test for heterogeneity between the studies is shown under the meta-analysis. The p value associated with the chi-square value is 0.0001, indicating that there is heterogeneity among the four studies.

It is important that reviewers try to explain heterogeneity among the studies. Heterogeneity may be due to the studies being conducted on different groups of patients, using different interventions (possibly different doses). In the GTR review, the heterogeneity among the four studies was investigated using several factors, including whether the patients underwent maintenance more than three times per month or not. This may be done by looking at subgroups of 'similar studies' to see whether the studies within each subgroup are homogeneous and the differences between studies are explained by differences between subgroups. Heterogeneity may also be investigated by using meta-regression. This involves multivariate, meta-analytic techniques, such as logistic regression, which is used to explore the relationship between the study characteristics (for example, allocation concealment, baseline risk, timing of the intervention), and study results (the magnitude of effect observed in each study) in a systematic review (Cochrane Library, Issue 1, 2001).

When heterogeneity is present, the reviewers must think hard about going ahead with the meta-analysis summary. Although it does not solve the problem of heterogeneity, if it is decided to continue with the data summary it may be wise to use a random effects model for combining the data rather than the conventional fixed effects model. A fixed effects model assumes that all the studies are estimating the same treatment effect, whether this is an odds ratio, a relative risk or a mean difference. A random effects model, however, does not make this assumption. It assumes that every study is estimating a different value, and that the random effects pooled estimate is simply averaging this out over the studies included. This means that in general the 95% confidence interval for the random effects model will be wider than that for the fixed effects model. The random effects model estimate was used in the Cochrane review for GTR and the overall weighted mean difference in the change in attachment from the ten studies was 1.11, with the 95% confidence interval from 0.63 to 1.59. The results for the fixed effects model estimate is mean attachment change 1.05, with 95% confidence interval from 0.81 to 1.28.

A random effects model was also used for the meta-analysis shown in Figure 5.1, and this gave a relative risk of 0.36 (95% CI: 0.19, 0.69) compared with the relative risk of 0.36, but narrower 95% confidence interval from 0.24 to 0.54, shown for the fixed effects model.

Publication bias

Publication bias is a bias in the published literature, where the publication of research depends on the nature and direction of the study results. Studies in which an intervention is not found to be effective are sometimes not published. Because of this, systematic reviews that fail to include unpublished studies may overestimate the true effect of an intervention (definition from the Cochrane Library). In order to try to control for publication bias, it is important that reviewers try to locate any unpublished studies. Statistical methods are available to detect publication bias, and they may be useful if there are a reasonable number of studies in the review (e.g. >15); when the number of studies is low it is difficult to detect publication bias statistically. Another way of visually examining for publication bias is the use of a funnel plot, which is a graph plotting sample size against effect size (Figure 5.3a). If publication bias is present, then there will be fewer non-significant small studies than there should be, leaving a gap in the 'funnel' shape of the graph (Figure 5.3b).

Sensitivity analysis

A sensitivity analysis is conduced to see how robust the overall summary statistic is. Frequently the meta-analysis is repeated to include the good quality studies only. The results of this are then compared with the

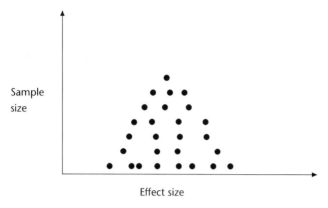

Figure 5.3(a) *Hypothetical symmetrical funnel plot of effect size versus sample size in the absence of bias.*

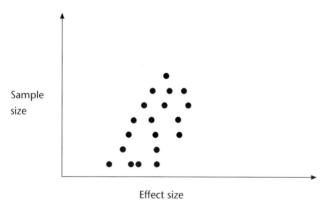

Figure 5.3(b) *Hypothetical asymmetrical plot of effect size versus sample size in the presence of publication bias.*

overall results. If the effect size is similar then this suggests that the overall result is robust. If the treatment effect is smaller for this group of high quality studies, this will weaken the interpretation of the overall effect size and may be cause for concern.

Subgroup analysis

Wherever possible, any hypotheses about potential subgroups (i.e. different age groups, males and females, different levels of fluoride, deciduous and permanent dentition, pockets >6 mm) should be stated a priori (in the protocol for the review). The number of planned subgroup analyses should be kept to a minimum to avoid spurious findings. Where there is significant heterogeneity in the results and no subgroup analysis has been stated a priori, subgroup analysis may be used, but the results should be interpreted with caution. Readers should be informed that the subgroup analysis was done because of the significant heterogeneity found, not because of an a priori hypothesis.

Specific problems with the data in dentistry

As the data from sites and teeth within a patient's mouth cannot be considered independent, this needs to be addressed in the analysis of many dental studies. Frequently the analysis has been conducted assuming the sites/teeth are independent and reviewers will then have to exclude these studies from the meta-analysis, unless they are able to obtain the raw data or the correct analysis from the study investigators.

Dental studies are frequently designed as crossover studies where, for example, half the patients are randomly allocated to receive mouth rinse A first, followed by mouth rinse B, while the other patients receive mouth rinse B followed by A. If correctly conducted, these studies may be combined with parallel group studies also investigating the relative efficacy of mouth rinses A and B. It is important to determine whether there is any carryover effect in the crossover studies before they are included in the meta-analysis.

Studies with a split-mouth design, where sites or teeth within the mouth are randomly allocated to the two interventions, are similar to crossover studies. These may also be combined with conventional parallel group studies where the patients are randomized to study groups. An example of this is the combining of these two study types in the guided tissue regeneration review (GTR).[11]

Sometimes the standard deviations are not given in the study reports. This is more of a problem in change studies (comparing the changes in disease from baseline), crossover and split-mouth studies, where the standard deviation of difference measurements is needed. Reviewers need to write to authors for the information and if this cannot be obtained they either estimate the values, or exclude the studies from the meta-analysis.

Statistical Software

The Cochrane Collaboration software (Review Manager software, RevMan 4.1) is readily available to everyone and may be down-loaded from the Internet from the Collaboration website http://www.cochrane.org/. The package contains a statistical element called Metaview, which may be used to conduct a meta-analysis. A more sophisticated analysis may be conducted using STATA software http://www.stata.com/ in which several statisticians working in this field have written specific procedures (ado files) for testing for publication bias, for heterogeneity and for carrying out a meta-regression. There are also other commercial packages dedicated to meta-analysis and there is an excellent discussion on these in two chapters of a recently published book on systematic reviews.[16,17]

References

1. Glass GV, Primary, secondary and meta-analysis of research, *Educ Res* (1976) 5:3–8.
2. Last JM, *A Dictionary of Epidemiology*, (Oxford University Press: New York, 1995).
3. Ebrahim S, Number needed to treat derived from meta-analyses: pitfalls and cautions. In: Egger M, Davey Smith G, Altman DG, eds, *Systematic Reviews* (BMJ Publishing Group: London, 2001) 386–399.
4. Clarkson JE, Worthington HV, Eden OB, Interventions for preventing oral

mucositis or oral candidiasis for patients with cancer receiving chemotherapy (excluding head and neck cancer) (Cochrane Review). *The Cochrane Library* Update Software 2000(1). http://www.update-software.com/cochrane

5. Bodey GP, Samonis G, Rolston K, Prophylaxis of candidiasis in cancer patients, *Seminars in Oncology* (1990) **17**(3):24–28.

6. Brincker H, Prevention of mycosis in granulocytopenic patients with prophylactic ketoconazole treatment, *Mykosen* (1983) **26**(5):242–247.

7. Caselli D, Arico M, Michelone G, Cavanna C, Nespoli L, Burgio GR, Antifungal chemoprophylaxis in cancer children: a prospective randomized controlled study, *Microbiologica* (1990) **13**:347–351.

8. Chandrasekar PH, Gatny CM, The effect of fluconazole prophylaxis on fungal colonisation in neutopenic cancer patients. Bone Marrow Transplantation Team, *J Antimicrob Chemother* (1994) **33**:309–318.

9. Palmblad J, Lonnqvist B, Carisson B, Grimfors G, Jarnmark M, Lerner R et al, Oral ketoconazole prophylaxis for Candida infections during induction therapy for acute leukaemia in adults: more bacteraemias, *J Intern Med* (1992) **231**:363–370.

10. Winston DJ, Chandrasekar PH, Lazarus HM, Goodman JL, Silber JL, Horowitz H et al., Fluconazole prophylaxis of fungal infections in patients with acute leukemia: results of a randomized placebo-controlled double-blind, multicenter trial, *Ann Intern Med* (1993) **118**:495–503.

11. Needleman IG, Giedrys-Leeper E, Tucker RJ et al, Guided tissue regeneration for periodontal infra-bony defects (Cochrane Review). The Cochrane Library, Update Software 2001(2). http://www.update-software.com/cochrane

12. Cortellini P, Pini Prato G, Tonetti M, Periodontal regeneration of human intrabony defects with titanium reinforced membranes. A controlled clinical trial, *J Periodontol* (1995) **66**(9):797–803.

13. Cortellini P, Pini Prato G, Tonetti M, Periodontal regeneration of human intrabony defects with bioresorbable membranes. A controlled clinical trial, *J Periodontol* (1996) **67**(3):217–223.

14. Mayfield L, Soderholm G, Hallstrom H, Kullendorff B, Edwardsson S, Bratthal G et al., Guided tissue regeneration for the treatment of intraosseous defects using a bioabsorbable membrane. A controlled clinical study, *J Clin Periodontol* (1998) **25**(7):585–595.

15. Tonetti MS, Cortellini P, Suvan JE, Adriaens P, Baldi C, Dubravec D et al., Generalizability of the added benefits of guided tissue regeneration in the treatment of deep intrabony defects. Evaluation in a multi-center randomized controlled clinical trial, *J Periodontol* (1998) **69**(11):1183–1192.

16. Sterne JAC, Egger M, Sutton AJ, Meta-analysis software, In: Egger M, Davey Smith G, Altman DG, eds, *Systematic reviews* (BMJ Publishing Group: London, 2001) 336–346.

17. Sterne JAC, Bradburn MJ, Egger M, Meta-analysis in Stata™, In: Egger M, Davey Smith G, Altman DG, eds, *Systematic reviews* (BMJ Publishing Group: London, 2001) 347–372.

chapter 6

The Cochrane Collaboration and its relevance to dentistry

Emma Tavender and Bill Shaw

It is surely a great criticism of our profession that we have not organized a critical summary, by specialty or subspecialty, updated periodically, of all relevant randomized controlled trials' (Archie Cochrane).[1]

Background

In 1972, Archie Cochrane, a British epidemiologist, published his influential book *Effectiveness and Efficiency: Random Reflections on Health Services*.[1] He drew attention to the great collective ignorance within the medical profession about the effects of health care and emphasized the importance of randomized controlled trials (RCTs) in guiding healthcare decisions. Trials must be properly designed, conducted, analyzed and reported. The results of these trials must then be assembled in systematic, up-to-date and accessible reviews.[2-4] Decision makers must take the results of these reviews into account and finally, based on these decisions, there must be effective systems to audit how well local or national guidelines for health care are followed.[5] If this is not done, important effects of health care (good and bad) will not be identified promptly, and people using the health services will be ill served as a result.[6] Without up-to-date systematic reviews of previous research, plans for new research will not be well informed. As a result, researchers and funding bodies will miss promising leads, and embark on studies asking questions that have already been answered.[6]

Systematic reviews may help to prevent treatments from being endorsed long after evidence from trials has concluded that they are useless or even harmful. Conversely they can help to shorten the time period between medical research discoveries and the implementation of effective treatment strategies. For example, if a systematic review of RCTs involving a short course of corticosteroids given to mothers about to give birth prematurely had been conducted in the 1980s, it would have shown that the corticosteroids substantially reduced the risk of neonatal morbidity and death.[7] Failure to conduct and apply a systematic review of the trials available resulted in the unnecessary suffering of tens of thousands of babies in addition to the increased costs of medical treatment for these babies.[8]

The Cochrane Collaboration

In response to Cochrane's call for up-to-date systematic reviews, the Cochrane Collaboration was established in 1992, under a National Health Service Research and Development initiative with the UK centre based in Oxford. The Cochrane Collaboration has now grown into an international organization with 15 centres established throughout the world. Its aims are to help clinicians, researchers, purchasers and patients to make well-informed decisions about health care by preparing, maintaining and promoting the accessibility of systematic reviews of the effects of health care interventions. The Cochrane Collaboration is guided by ten key principles (Box 6.1).

The core work of the Collaboration is carried out by 50 international Collaborative Review Groups (CRGs), who have the responsibility of preparing and maintaining Cochrane reviews. The members of these groups: healthcare professionals, researchers, consumers and others, share an interest in ensuring the availability of reliable, up-to-date evidence relevant to the prevention, treatment and rehabilitation of a particular health

Box 6.1 Principles of the Cochrane Collaboration

■ **Collaboration . . .**
by internally and externally fostering good communications, open decision-making and teamwork.

■ **Building on the enthusiasm of individuals . . .**
by involving and supporting people of different skills and backgrounds.

■ **Avoiding duplication . . .**
by good management and co-ordination to maximize economy of effort.

■ **Minimizing bias . . .**
through a variety of approaches such as scientific rigour, ensuring broad participation, and avoiding conflicts of interest.

■ **Keeping up to date . . .**
by a commitment to ensure that Cochrane Reviews are maintained through identification and incorporation of new evidence.

■ **Striving for relevance . . .**
by promoting the assessment of health care interventions using outcomes that matter to people making choices in health care.

■ **Promoting access . . .**
by wide dissemination of the outputs of the Collaboration, taking advantage of strategic alliances, and by promoting appropriate prices, content and media to meet the needs of users worldwide.

■ **Ensuring quality . . .**
by being open and responsive to criticism, applying advances in methodology, and developing systems for quality improvement.

■ **Continuity . . .**
by ensuring that responsiblity for reviews, editorial processes, and key functions is maintained and renewed.

■ **Enabling wide participation . . .**
in the work of the collaboration by reducing barriers to contributing and by encouraging diversity

problem or group of problems.[9] One such group is the Cochrane Oral Health Group, which is discussed in more detail in Chapter 7.

The work of the CRGs is supported and co-ordinated by 15 Cochrane Centres around the world. It is their responsibility to provide guidance, training and support for the entities and individual contributors within the geographical area for which they are responsible.

The methods which reviewers use to prepare systematic reviews draw on the experience of various Cochrane methods working groups. Methodologists within these methods working groups promote and support relevant empirical methodological research and help to improve the validity and precision of the systematic reviews.[9,10]

Cochrane fields/networks are groups of people with a healthcare interest that spans a number of CRGs. This interest could be the setting of care (for example, primary care), the type of consumer (for example, child health), the type of provider (nurses) or the type of intervention (vaccines). Cochrane fields ensure that the priorities and perspectives of their particular subject area are reflected in the work of the CRGs, they comment on systematic reviews within their particular subject area and liaise with relevant agencies and organizations. In addition, fields are involved in hand searching specialist journals and contributing to the Cochrane Controlled Trials Register, described below and in Chapter 2.

The Consumer Network was established to reflect consumer interests within the Cochrane Collaboration. Consumers participate throughout most of the organization. Collaborative Review Groups, Centres and Fields all seek input and feedback from consumers, which is considered essential in order to fulfil the goals of the Cochrane Collaboration.

The Cochrane Library

The main product of the Cochrane Collaboration is the Cochrane Database of Systematic Reviews that forms part of the Cochrane Library, a quarterly electronic publication. The Cochrane Library may be purchased on CD-ROM or subscribed to on the Internet directly from the publisher (Update Software: Oxford, UK).

There are several databases included in the Cochrane Library.

- **The Cochrane Database of Systematic Reviews** is a collection of regularly updated systematic reviews of the effects of health care and maintained by the Cochrane Collaboration.
- **The Cochrane Controlled Trials Register (CCTR)** is a bibliographic database of controlled trials which includes references downloaded from MEDLINE, EMBASE, and trials identified as part of the Collaboration's international effort to hand search the world's journals and create an unbiased source of data for systematic reviews.[10]
- **Database of Abstracts of Reviews of Effectiveness (DARE)** includes structured abstracts of non-Cochrane systematic reviews. The NHS Centre for Reviews and Dissemination (CRD) in York critically appraises the reviews, prepares the structured abstracts and maintains the DARE database.
- **Cochrane Review Methodology Database** is a bibliography of articles on the science of research synthesis.
- **Health Technology Assessment Database (HTA)** is compiled by the NHS Centre for Reviews and Dissemination and was formerly part of the Database of Abstracts of Reviews of Effectiveness. This database contains information on healthcare technology assessments.
- **NHS Economic Evaluation Database (NHS EED)** is a companion to the CRD Database of Abstracts of Reviews of Effectiveness (DARE). It is a register of published economic evaluations of healthcare interventions.

Cochrane systematic reviews – how different are they from traditional systematic reviews?

The systematic review is based on an explicit and rigorous process that includes a clear description of the objectives, explicit criteria for including studies, an explicit description of why relevant studies have not been considered, extraction of data, pooling of data from similar studies (meta-analysis), description of results, drawing appropriate conclusions and discussing implications for clinical practice and future research.[11]

As Cochrane emphasized, systematic reviews of RCTs must be kept up to date and take into account new evidence so that important effects of health care will be identified promptly. As Cochrane systematic reviews are in electronic format, reviewers are able to update and modify their reviews in response to new evidence and comments and criticisms from readers. The Cochrane Criticisms Editor, an electronic facility included in the Cochrane Library, is for the delivery of comments on Cochrane reviews to authors and editors.[12] The quality of reviews is therefore enhanced by means of a system that not only reflects the emergence of new data but also responds to valid criticisms from whatever source.

Cochrane reviews are updated more frequently than their paper-based counterparts, with a policy that reviews should be updated within 2 years of publication and then at least every 2 years thereafter.[13] There are also major differences between the peer review process of the Cochrane Collaboration and that of the paper-based journals. There are several levels to the peer review process of the Collaboration, including the assessment of protocols by editors and reviewers and the evaluation of the reviews methodology and content by potential users/consumers.[12] It has been suggested that due to the existence of this thorough refereeing process, Cochrane reviews are less prone to bias than systematic reviews or meta-analyses published in paper-based journals.[14]

Progress to date

The Cochrane Collaboration has only been in existence for ten years; however, it has achieved a great deal in this short time span. With the release of Issue 2, April 2002 of the Cochrane Library there are 1,350 Cochrane systematic reviews and 1,055 protocols published, with approximately 340,000 references to reports of trials on CCTR. Although not all healthcare topics have been covered by Cochrane systematic reviews, the organization is continually growing and has approximately 16,000 contributors around the world. With the continued enthusiasm and goodwill of contributors it is envisaged that the number of topics covered will increase, making the Cochrane Library an invaluable resource for healthcare providers, researchers and policy makers.

What relevance has the Cochrane Collaboration to dentistry?

Needless to say, up-to-date systematic reviews are as essential to the successful provision of oral health care and policy. Many dentists work in relative isolation, with no hope of critically evaluating the thousands of journal articles published every year in the oral health field, nor of verifying the claims of those advocating novel interventions or materials. Equally, in specialist fields, there is huge diversity in practices, and on the basis of the reviews already performed (see Chapter 7), limited evidence for the effectiveness of common interventions.

Archie Cochrane's challenge to the providers of medical care applies with equal force to those of us in the field of oral health.

References

1. Cochrane AL, *Effectiveness and Efficiency: Random Reflections on Health Services*, (Nuffield Provincial Hospitals Trust: London, 1972). Reprinted for the Nuffield Trust (Royal Society of Medical Press: London, 1999).
2. Chalmers I, Improving the quality and dissemination of reviews of clinical research. In: Lock S, ed, *The Future of Medical Journals*, (BMJ Publishing Group: London, 1991) 127–146.
3. Mulrow CD, The medical review article: state of the science, *Ann Intern Med* (1987) **106**:485–488.
4. Haynes RB, Clinical review articles, *BMJ* (1991) 304:330–331.
5. Chalmers I, Dickersin K, Chalmers TC, Getting to grips with Archie Cochrane's agenda, *BMJ* (1992) **305**:786–788.
6. Chalmers I, The Cochrane Collaboration: preparing, maintaining, and disseminating systematic reviews of the effects of health care. *Ann NY Acad Sci* (1993) **703**:156–163.
7. Crowley P, Chalmers I, Keirse MJNC, The effects of corticosteroid administration before preterm delivery: an overview of the evidence from controlled trials, *Br J Obstet Gynaecol* (1990) **97**:11–25.
8. Mugford M, Poercy J, Chalmers I, Cost implications of different approaches to the prevention of respiratory distress syndrome, *Arch Dis Child* (1991) **66**: 757–764.

9. Alderson P, The Cochrane Collaboration: an introduction, *Evidence-Based Dentistry* (1998) **1**:25–26.
10. Antes G, Oxman AD, The Cochrane Collaboration in the 20th century. In: Egger M, Davey Smith G, Altman DG, eds, *Systematic Reviews in Health Care. Meta-analysis in Context*, 3rd edn (BMJ Publishing Group: London, 2001) 447–458.
11. Neilson JP, Levene MI, The Cochrane Collaboration: progress in perinatal medicine, *Arch Dis Child Fetal Neonatal Ed* (1997) **77**:176F–177F.
12. Jadad AR, Haynes RB, The Cochrane Collaboration: advances and challenges in improving evidence-based decision making, *Med Decis Making* (1998) **279**: 611–614.
13. Jadad AR, Cook DJ, Jones A et al, Methodology and reports of systematic reviews and meta-analyses: a comparison of Cochrane reviews with articles published in paper-based journals, *JAMA* (1998) **280**:278–280.
14. Egger M, Davey Smith G, Schneider M et al, Bias in meta-analysis detected by a simple, graphical test, *BMJ* (1997) **315**:629–634.

chapter 7

Systematic reviews in dentistry: the role of the Cochrane Oral Health Group

Helen Worthington and Jan Clarkson

Introduction

To help people make well-informed decisions about health care, it is important that systematic summaries of current best evidence are available. In dentistry, as in other healthcare professions, to achieve this we need to overcome certain challenges. For the profession to rely on non-systematic reviews, out-of-date summaries and the occasional systematic summary, or to delay a decision until an up-to-date summary has been completed, is not acceptable – though it is common practice today. In this chapter we would like to discuss the process of conducting a Cochrane review and the role of the Oral Health Group.

The challenges faced by those with the desire to make high quality summaries of evidence available have been categorized as ethical, social, logistical and methodological.[1] To maximize the effort and minimize the duplication of people conducting reviews, both the ethical and social challenges of how we work and work together need to be addressed. It is pointless for multiple teams to undertake the same comprehensive review and for this to be repeated at a later date. Logistical issues include the identification of all the evidence and the update of reviews, whilst methodological challenges include establishing guidance for what types of studies should be included and how these can be combined and interpreted.

Cochrane Library

As a source of systematic reviews 'The Cochrane Database of Systematic Reviews', in the Cochrane Library comprises more than 1,300 reviews of healthcare interventions, usually only including randomized controlled trials (RCTs) or controlled clinical trials (CCTs). Empirical research indicates that Cochrane Systematic Reviews are, on average, of higher quality than those published in journals.[2] This does not mean that they cannot be improved upon.[3] The Cochrane Oral Health Group (OHG) is one of 50 Cochrane review groups, each looking at a disease area. The OHG was initiated in New England (USA) by Alexia Antczak-Bouckoms, in 1994 and moved to Manchester (UK) in 1996, securing NHS funding for the editorial base in 1997. Since then progress has been excellent; there are now 10 reviews, 29 protocols and 40 titles registered. The reviews conducted by the Cochrane Oral Health Group may be accessed in the Cochrane Library. They are listed on the OHG website: http://www.cochrane-oral.man.ac.uk and the abstracts may be viewed on http://www.cochrane.org.

A growing comprehensive source of non-Cochrane systematic reviews in health care, including dentistry, is available. The Database of Abstracts of Reviews of Effectiveness (DARE) includes high quality systematic research reviews (published since 1994 in journals indexed in the following electronic databases: Current Contents Clinical Medline, MEDLINE, CINAHL, CLINICAL, ERIC, Biosis, Allied and Alternative Medicine, PsycINFO) of the effectiveness of healthcare interventions. DARE has been compiled by the NHS Centre for Reviews and Dissemination (CRD) at York University. A structured abstract written by CRD reviewers is given for each review, along with the CRD commentary on the quality of the review. About 65 systematic reviews have been identified in the oral health area, of which around 20 concerned pain control for dental and other surgical procedures. The remainder includes a range of topics including periodontics, caries, oral medicine, oral maxillofacial surgery, restorative dentistry, temporomandibular disorders, orthodontics, oral health promotion and sleep apnoea. The majority of the systematic reviews focused on the treatment of a disease or disorder with the others covering prevention, diagnosis and adverse events.

Continual updates can be viewed on the CRD website http://www.york.ac.uk/inst/crd/welcome.htm or in the Cochrane Library. An up-to-date list of these reviews is also given on the Oral Health Group website.

Oral Health Group

The scope of the OHG is oral health, broadly conceived to include the prevention, treatment and rehabilitation of oral, dental and craniofacial diseases and disorders. One of the initial logistical challenges has been to identify all the evidence. The OHG Specialized Register is a database of trials related to the group; it currently includes over 13,000 randomized controlled trials, controlled clinical trials and associated material such as conference proceedings and research abstracts. The OHG trials search co-ordinator continually updates the register, and organizes the hand searching of the dental literature. This consists of going through each journal page by page, identifying any reports of possible trials. Currently 42 dental journals have/are being searched by 11 hand searchers. This register is the most comprehensive register of RCTs in dentistry and is a good place to search if conducting a review including RCTs. Trial reports included in the OHG specialized register will also be included in the Cochrane Controlled Trials Register (CCTR) in the Cochrane Library, although this may involve a 6-month delay.[2] The Cochrane Controlled Trials Register contains 340,000 reports of trials in medicine overall and is a useful place to begin a more general search for trials.

For a systematic review to be comprehensive, all the evidence needs to be available. It is important to identify unpublished research, so the

OHG has recently contacted all the major oral pharmaceutical companies asking for their help in locating such trials within the oral health field. The responses received so far have been very positive, though not as comprehensive as Glaxo Wellcome and Schering Healthcare. These two companies are currently working with Dr Iain Chalmers of the UK Cochrane Centre to document their unpublished clinical trials in a register to be made available to the medical community. As prospective registration of research becomes more widely implemented, the role of the OHG in identifying trials should diminish dramatically, but for now there is still a considerable way to go.

Editorial process for conducting a review

The OHG group has a worldwide list of members, a panel of referees and a list of potential reviewers. The ethical challenge of building on enthusiasm, whilst avoiding duplication and minimizing bias, can in part be addressed by effective communication. The first part of the editorial process of the OHG is to register a title with the group (Figure 7.1). Cochrane titles take a specific format as follows: (intervention) for (disease) in (patient group). At this stage the OHG can check that there is no overlap with other registered reviews. It is also helpful to check whether there is another similar review on the DARE database. As with any research the most important part is asking the right question(s). The OHG tries to avoid reviewers asking too big a question, as the resulting reviews are difficult to conduct, use and maintain. One person alone cannot produce a review; not only is it difficult, but it can lead to bias, so at this stage we pull together a team of people willing to collaborate. One of the social challenges confronting us is to accommodate diversity by bringing together people from different backgrounds, cultures and different types of expertise. Multidisciplinary teams are best, comprising clinical specialists, general dentists/nurses/hygienists and methodologists. We have successfully accommodated the interests of enthusiastic individuals with overlapping interests and avoided any monopolizing of areas. The unexpected outcome has been for indi-

Register titles
Prepare protocol:
- Background
- Objectives
- Criteria for including studies in the review:
  o Types of studies
  o Types of participants
  o Types of interventions
  o Types of outcomes
- Search strategy for identification of studies
- Methods of the review:
  o Selection of studies
  o Decisions about eligibility
  o Data extraction
  o Quality assessment
  o Data synthesis
Protocol goes out for internal and external review
Protocol appears in Cochrane Library
Conduct search
Select studies
Extract data
Conduct quality assessment of studies
Data synthesis
Write completed review:
- Consumer synopsis
- Implications for practice
- Implications for research
Review goes out for internal and external review
Review appears in Cochrane Library
Review is updated every 2 years

Figure 7.1 *The reviewing process for the Cochrane Oral Health Group.*

viduals to experience something of greater significance than purely working on a review.

Once a title is registered, the reviewers write a protocol for the review. This can be the hardest part of a review and it is helpful for inexperienced reviewers to attend a protocol workshop, conducted by the

Cochrane Centres. The OHG provide assistance with the protocol and we usually expect that it be completed within 6–9 months. The background section contains clear and concise details outlining the clinical problem. The objectives are stated along with the criteria for considering studies for inclusion in the review. This includes details of the types of studies, participants, interventions and outcomes. It is important to state whether the intervention is being compared with a placebo or no treatment control, or with another intervention.

The protocol will also state the search strategy to be used. It is usual to carry out the search strategy on at least two electronic databases. Usually we do not restrict the search to the English language as this could introduce bias. The OHG will try to ensure that reports of studies in other languages are translated, or the relevant data extracted by Cochrane collaborators from across the world. Reviewers also need to consider how they are going to access any unpublished studies. This process necessitates considerable resource and it is important for social inclusion that people from low to middle-income countries have the opportunity to participate in the collaboration. It is an accolade to our profession that one of the notable challengers of conventional dental practice, Aubrey Sheiham, has made available the Sheiham Public Health and Primary Care Scholarship which supports travel, IT and training in Cochrane systematic reviews for people from developing countries.

It is our ambition to limit bias by making the methods and assumptions underlying a review explicit and as clear as possible. The method section of the review protocol therefore includes details about how the studies are to be selected, the eligibility criteria and the data extraction. These are usually done independently, in duplicate, by at least two separate reviewers. The quality assessment is carried out in the same way and the findings of the two reviewers compared, to assess the level of agreement. Details of the data synthesis are also included in the protocol. It is important that issues relating to heterogeneity and subgroup analysis are determined before the data are collected. A sensitivity analysis that includes the good quality studies is usually proposed.

Whilst the use of data synthesis in the form of a meta-analysis has been used for almost a century, the science of systematically reviewing medical research is young. Consequently, considerable effort is being given to the methodological aspects of this type of research. The design of dental research presents some particular challenges such as how to handle data from split-mouth and crossover studies. Deciding what types of study to include in a review also presents a challenge. The argument for restricting study design to RCTs has a logical and empirical basis, however, it may sometimes be appropriate to conduct reviews of other types of studies. The OHG is currently putting systems in place for decision rules to include or exclude different types of studies depending upon the questions being asked.

Once the protocol has been completed it is sent out for both internal (by the OHG editorial team) and external peer review. Once it has been through this process and all the referees' comments have been addressed, it is entered into the Cochrane Library. The reviewers can now get down to conducting the review along the lines laid down in the protocol. This usually takes between 12 and 18 months.

The final review contains a synopsis for consumers (Figure 7.2), and the review's conclusions include implications for practice and for research. It is not a function of the review to make treatment recommendations, but to present a summary of the evidence. Before the review is included in the Cochrane Library it goes out for peer review, and our experience has been that members of the Cochrane Collaboration provide the most constructive criticisms we have encountered. Reviewers understand before they conduct a Cochrane review that once the review appears on the Library, they are committed to update the review every two years. It is a logistical challenge to ensure this happens. Maintaining the enthusiasm of a review team is one thing, but the importance of assuring academic recognition for maintenance after the initial publication also needs to be recognized.

More often than not, healthcare interventions have some beneficial effects, some harmful effects and costs associated with them. There is always some degree of uncertainty about all of these and the people making decisions or recommendations need information that is as explicit as possible. It is important that reviews are conducted to answer important questions and that might be in an area where there is little

Interventions for preventing oral mucositis or oral candidiasis for patients with cancer receiving chemotherapy (excluding head and neck cancer)

Clarkson JE, Worthington HV, Eden OB (January 2000)

Synopsis: Sucking ice chips appears to prevent mouth ulcers caused by chemotherapy for cancer, and some anti-fungal drugs can prevent oral thrush associated with chemotherapy.

Chemotherapy for cancer (including bone marrow transplant) can cause severe ulcers and fungal infections (thrush) in the mouth. These can cause discomfort, pain, difficulties in eating, and a longer stay in hospital. Different strategies are used to try and prevent these conditions. These include taking tablets, using a mouthwash or sucking ice chips, before and during the cancer treatment. The review found that sucking ice chips prevented ulcers, and taking anti-fungal tablets can prevent fungal infections.

Interventions for treating oral lichen planus

Chan ES-Y, Thornhill M, Zakrzewska J (April 1999)

Synopsis: Weak evidence for effectiveness of therapies for oral lichen planus

Oral lichen planus is a longterm, painful, disease of ulcers on the mouth lining of unknown cause. There is no cure and treatment is given to reduce the pain. Many therapies have been tried but this review found that only a few had ever been compared against placebo and no agent's effectiveness had been confirmed in separate studies. All studies reported that treatment was effective but the uncertainty was high because of the small patient numbers. Toxic side-effects were only seen in agents taken internally (systemic) as opposed to those applied to the mouth surface.

Orthodontic treatment for posterior crossbites

Harrison JE, Ashby D (January 2001)

Synopsis: Early treatment of posterior crossbites appears to prevent them from being passed on to the adult dentition. However, this is only based on data from two small studies.

'Posterior crossbite' occurs when the top back teeth bite inside the bottom back teeth. It is unclear what causes posterior crossbites and they may develop or improve at any time from when the baby teeth come into the mouth to when the adult teeth come through. If they affect one side of the mouth the lower jaw may need to move to one side to allow the back teeth to meet together. This movement may have long-term effects on the growth of the teeth and jaws. Several treatments have been used to correct posterior crossbites and stop this abnormal movement.

Potassium nitrate toothpaste for dentine hypersensitivity
Poulsen S, Errboe M, Hovgaard O, Worthington HW (April 2001)
Synopsis: There is not enough evidence to show that potassium nitrate toothpaste helps reduce dental hypersensitivity.

Dentine hypersensitivity is a sharp, sudden pain arising when teeth are exposed to touch or hot and cold foods. If dental disease is not the cause of the pain, toothpastes containing potassium nitrate are sometimes used to reduce teeth sensitivity. The review of trials found there was not enough evidence to show that potassium nitrate is effective in desensitising teeth. More research is needed.

Interventions for the treatment of burning mouth syndrome
Zakrzewska JM, Glenny AM, Forssell H (September 2001)
Synopsis: Not enough evidence exists to show the effect of pain-killers, vitamins, hormones, anti-depressants for 'burning mouth syndrome' but there is some evidence that learning to cope with the disorder may help.

A burning sensation on the lips, tongue or within the mouth is called 'burning mouth syndrome' when the cause is unknown and it is not a symptom of another disease. Other symptoms include dryness and altered taste, and it is common in people with anxiety, depression and personality disorders. Women after menopause are at highest risk of this syndrome. Pain-killers, vitamin supplements, hormone therapies, and anti-depressants have all been tried as possible cures. This review did not find enough evidence to show their effects. Treatments designed to help people cope with the discomfort may be beneficial. More research is needed.

Interventions for treating oral candidiasis for patients with cancer receiving treatment
Clarkson JE, Worthington HV, Eden OB (February 2002)
Synopsis: The anti-fungal drugs ketoconazole and clotrimazole might be able to cure oral thrush caused by cancer treatment.
Cancer treatment can lead to severe fungal infections (candidiasis, called thrush) in the mouth. This can cause pain, difficulties in eating and longer hospital stays. Infection can sometimes spread through the body and become life-threatening. Different drugs are used to try and relieve candidiasis. There is weak evidence that some of the antifungal drugs may cure fungal infections in the mouth for people with cancer. It may be that drugs like keoconazole and clotrimazole, which are absorbed fully (or partially) through the gastrointestinal

tract, are more effective than those which are not absorbed (like nystatin), but more research is needed.

Interventions for treating oral mucositis for patients with cancer receiving treatment

Worthington HV, Clarkson JE, Eden OB (February 2002)

Synopsis: Using an allopurinol mouthwash or vitamin E may relieve or cure ulcers caused by cancer treatment.

Treatments for cancer can cause severe ulcers (sores) in the mouth. These can be painful and slow recovery. Options include taking tablets, using a mouthwash, or different ways of coping, before and during the cancer treatment. The review found weak and unreliable evidence that using an allopurinol mouthwash or vitamin E may relieve or cure the ulcers. Morphine can control the pain. Although using morphine automatically, or self-controlled use, provide similar relief, people use less morphine when they are controlling it themselves.

Interventions for treating oral leukoplakia

Lodi G, Sardella A, Bez C, Demarosi F, Carrassi A. (February 2002)

Synopsis: No evidence exists from trials to show how to prevent leukoplakia in the mouth becoming malignant.

Oral leukoplakia is a thickened white patch formed in the mouth lining that cannot be rubbed off. Leukoplakia is a lesion that sometimes becomes cancerous (a tumour that invades and destroys tissue, then spreads to other areas). Preventing this change is critical, since survival rates of more than five years after diagnosis with oral cancer are low. Drugs, surgery and other therapies have been tried. The review of trials compared several drugs such as bleomycin, vitamin A and beta carotene supplements and mixed tea. There was no evidence found to show the effects of these treatments. More research is needed.

Guided tissue regeneration for periodontal infra-bony defects

Needleman IG, Giedrys-Leeper E, Tucker RJ, Worthington HV (October 2001)

Synopsis: Current treatments for destructive periodontal (gum) disease are not able to restore damaged bone and connective tissue support for teeth. There are therefore limitations in treating patients with advanced disease. The surgical technique of guided tissue regeneration (GTR) may be able to achieve regeneration and therefore improve upon conventional surgical results. The results of this review have shown some advantage for GTR but with wide variations in the benefits achievable compared with conventional open flap surgery. We were unable to conclusively identify factors associated with more successful outcomes and we therefore recommend further research to address this issue.

Fluoride gels for preventing dental caries in children and adolescents
Marinho VCC, Higgins JPT, Logan S, Sheiham A (April 2002)
Synopsis: Using fluoride gels a few times a year would reduce tooth decay in many children, although more research is needed on possible adverse effects.
    Fluoride is a mineral that prevents tooth decay (dental caries). Since widespread use of fluoride toothpastes and water fluoridation, the value of additional fluoride has been questioned. Fluoride gels can be professionally or self-applied under supervision, at a frequency from once to several times a year. The review of trials found that fluoride gel can reduce tooth decay in children. As many as one in two children with high levels of tooth decay (and one in 24 with the lowest levels) would have less decay. However, more research is needed on adverse effects, as children often swallow gel during application.

Figure 7.2 Cochrane Oral Health Group Systematic Reviews (Cochrane Library Issue 2, 2002).

evidence. The reasons for identifying these are twofold, to make clear to people making the decisions what the evidence is, and to support the decisions of funding bodies and researchers to undertake new research. Involving consumers in this process in an effective rather than a token way is a challenge. After all, they are the ultimate beneficiaries of the work and the reason why we undertake this task.

We are aware that the reviews currently published through the OHG answer few of the questions asked by people making decisions about their oral health care, but the list of protocols demonstrates a commitment to continue to act and to act quickly (Figure 7.3). The challenges faced by those involved in synthesizing evidence in dentistry need to be

Combinations of topical fluorides (varnishes, gels, rinses, toothpastes) versus one topical fluoride for preventing dental caries in children and adolescents	VCC Marinho
Fluoride rinses for preventing dental caries in children and adolescents	VCC Marinho
Fluoride toothpastes for preventing dental caries in children and adolescents	VCC Marinho
Fluoride varnishes for preventing dental caries in children and adolescents	VCC Marinho
Glues for fixing dental braces onto teeth	NA Mandall
Interventions for maintaining health tissues around dental implants	M Esposito
Interventions for replacing missing teeth with or without osseointegrated implants	M Esposito
Manual versus powered toothbrushing for oral health	WC Shaw
One topical fluoride (varnishes, or gels, or rinses, or toothpastes) versus another for preventing dental caries in children and adolescents	VCC Marinho
Fluoride varnishes versus sealants for caries prevention	A Nordblad
Retention procedures for stabilising tooth position after treatment with orthodontic braces	SJ Littlewood
Topical fluoride (toothpastes, mouthrinses, gels or varnishes) for preventing dental caries in children and adolescents	VCC Marinho
Hyaluronate for treating temporomandibular joint disorders	S Zongdao
Conscious sedation for dental anxiety	P McGoldrick
Psychotherapy for dental anxiety	P McGoldrick
Pulp treatment for extensive decay in primary (milk) teeth	G Nadin

Feeding interventions for infants with cleft lip, cleft palate or cleft lip and palate	AM Glenny
Topical fluoride for treating dental caries	MA Ferreira de Oliveria
Orthodontic treatment for children with prominent upper front teeth	JE Harrison
Orthodontic treatment for children with prominent lower front teeth	JE Harrison
Orthodontic treatment for crowded teeth in children	JE Harrison
Ceramic inlays for restoring teeth	M Hayashi
Interventions for replacing missing teeth: bone augmentation techniques for dental implant treatment	P Coulthard
Interventions for replacing missing teeth: hyperbaric oxygen therapy for dental implant treatment	P Coulthard
Interventions for replacing missing teeth: pre-prosthetic surgery	P Coulthard
Interventions for replacing missing teeth: resin-bonded bridges and other restorations for the replacement of adult teeth	B Swift
Interventions for replacing missing teeth: surgical techniques for placing dental implants	P Coulthard
Pit and fissure sealants for preventing dental decay in the permanent teeth of children and adolescents	A Nordblad
Pit and fissure sealants versus varnishes for preventing dental decay in the permanent teeth of children and adolescents	A Hiiri
Stabilisation split therapy for temporomandibular pain dysfunction syndrome	MZ Al-Ani

Figure 7.3 Cochrane Oral Health Group Protocols
(Cochrane Library, Issue 2, 2002).

addressed by a wider group than the OHG at international level. For the OHG, our priority is nurturing the most precious resource we have: the many hard working people who are collaborating with us. Ultimately, dissemination of the synthesized evidence in a format which is digestible for the user, whether that be a patient, practitioner or policy maker, will determine how effective we are at improving the quality of dental health care.

References

1. Oxman, AD, The Cochrane Collaboration in the 20th century: Ten challenges and one reason why they must be met, In: Egger M, Davey Smith G, Altman DG, eds, *Systematic Reviews in Health Care: Meta-analysis in Context*, 3rd edn (BMJ Publishing Group: London, 2001) 459–473.
2. Jadad AR, Moher M, Browman GP, Booker L, Sigouin C, Fuentes M et al, Systematic reviews and meta-analysis on treatment of asthma: critical evaluation, *BMJ* (2000) **320**:537–540.
3. Olsen O, Middleton P, Ezzo J, Gotzsche PC, Hadhazy V, Herxheimer A, Kleijnen J, McIntosh M, Quality of Cochrane reviews: assessment of sample from 1998, *BMJ* (2001) **323**:829–832.

chapter 8

How are other levels of evidence being used?

Brian C Bonner

Karl Popper, widely acknowledged as the twentieth century's greatest philosopher of scientific method, advised us to 'Try to learn what people are discussing nowadays in science. Find out where difficulties arise and take an interest in disagreements. These are the questions which you should take up.'[1] The pursuit of good medical science must be guided by a no-lesser spirit of probing enquiry. There have been examples of established practice which have proved to be less than useful when put to rigorously controlled clinical trial. A report into *Unnecessary dental treatment*[2] was requested by the UK Minister of Health, as a result of concern expressed by the British Dental Association, Family Practitioner Committees and the public. In the provision of orthodontic treatment, for instance, it has been found that much inappropriate and ineffective treatment has been carried out. A study involving 1210 patients concluded that a high proportion of orthodontic patients showed no improvement after treatment. Analysing treatment according to the type of appliance used revealed no significant difference in standards between specialist orthodontists and general dental practitioners.[3] A more recent study, examining clinical outcome for children born with unilateral cleft lip and palate in the UK, found that only 58% of bone grafts that had been undertaken were successful.[4] Less than one-third of subjects had a good facial appearance as judged by a panel of experts, despite levels of patient and parent satisfaction being generally high. A previous study carried out at the University of North Carolina, USA, had concluded that 54% of 495 children interviewed, with cleft lip or cleft lip and palate, were very pleased with their appearance post surgery.[5]

The gold standard to inform evidence based practice is use of systematic review of multiple well designed, randomized, controlled trials. This is the type of evidence published by organizations such as the Cochrane Collaboration, as outlined in Chapter 6. However, in reality, the evidence available to dental practitioners ranges from this very high standard at one end of the spectrum, right through to evidence of doubtful value and misinformation at the other. The busy practitioner, though s/he may take an interest in following research, in practice only needs to know the conclusions that have been reached by those whose day-to-day business is the careful analysis of research findings. Practitioners need to make treatment decisions based on the best evidence and advice available to them, but have not the time, nor perhaps the experience, to read, assimilate, and draw conclusions from academic research papers. This chapter discusses some of the sources to which dental health professionals may turn for advice and information. Such sources are changeable by nature and, increasingly, new forms of delivery, such as on-line resources, are being explored.

The amount of material published on oral health, as with most other subjects of public interest, is considerable. A busy member of the dental team would never find the time to even read all that is available, let alone digest and appraise the content. Over the last several years, a number of publications have addressed this issue, with an attempt to provide 'potted' summaries and to reprint selected articles for the benefit of the people for whom they may be relevant. It started around 1995, when the *British Medical Journal* and the American College of Physicians began to publish *Evidence-Based Medicine*, subtitled *Linking Research to Practice*. The strategy employed was 'to screen over 50 journals for articles on diagnosis, prognosis, therapy, aetiology, quality of care, and health economics that are both relevant to medical practice and adhere to rigorous methodological standards for patient-based research'.[6] This was followed by related journals devoted to evidence based practice in other disciplines, including, three years later, *Evidence-Based Dentistry*, published by the British Dental Association. This publication aims to select '... those original and review articles whose results are most likely to be both true and useful'. The articles are summarized by acknow-ledged experts in the field in a 'value-added' form.

A slightly older, pamphlet-style publication, *Bandolier*, is published monthly and is available on the World Wide Web (WWW) at http://www.jr2.ox.ac.uk/bandolier/.

The impetus behind the creation of *Bandolier* was 'to find information about evidence of effectiveness (or lack of it), and to put it forward as simple "bullet-points" of those things that succeeded and those things that didn't'. The production of *Bandolier* was stimulated by a claim made by a general practitioner, perceived by the publication's founders to be improbable, that only seven things (in medicine) were known to be effect-ive. Information published in *Bandolier* was to come from systematic reviews of the medical literature, from *Effectiveness Bulletins* from York (see below), from randomized, controlled trials, and from high-quality case–control, cohort, or observational studies. 25,000 copies of *Bandolier* are currently distributed to general practitioners and the on-line version, hosted by the University of Oxford, provides full, free-of-charge, access-ible-to-all text. A new initiative in May 1999, from the same stable, was the parallel publication of *ImpAct*, which continued bi-monthly until funding was regrettably withdrawn in March 2001. The difference in emphasis between the two publications was that, whilst *Bandolier* concen-trated on collating and presenting high-quality evidence, *ImpAct*'s empha-sis was on the way in which the evidence could be used to improve standards of healthcare service to patients. *ImpAct* included reports from people who had led successful local initiatives and who were keen for others to learn from their experience, with contact details being given to allow articles to be followed up by interested parties.

The WWW has seen a staggering increase in the number of users in the industrialized world, and more and more people are now maturing in their use of the Web and discovering that it can be used for informa-tion retrieval as well as electronic mail. Many individuals and organ-izations provide health information on the Web as well as in print, with others publishing on the Web only. This 'on-line' information is mostly available to both the providers of care and to patients; in some instances, access is restricted to subscribers or registered users. Information available on the WWW encompasses a greater range of quality than that found in print and the healthcare professional needs to be careful that the provider is a reputable source.[7] Obtaining information from the WWW can, to the novice user, seem, initially, a daunting task. Catalogues and indices, generally supported by advertising revenues, are accessed through search engines. By entering the search word 'dental' into the *Google* search engine (http://www.google.com), the user is offered a choice of 3.75 million pages to browse (each reached by 'clicking' on the supplied links); 'oral health' generates half this number. Clearly, targeting the best available evidence from a choice such as this is a monumental task that few would seriously attempt.

A number of dental institutions and organizations have responded to this information overload by providing sites where visitors can link to a variety of useful information. A representative sample of these will be briefly outlined.

■ The NHS Centre for Reviews and Dissemination, at the University of York, UK, http://www.york.ac.uk/inst/crd/dissinfo.htm, commissions and undertakes systematic reviews, publishes Cochrane Collaboration systematic reviews, and publishes high-quality reviews undertaken elsewhere. Compared to general medicine, comparatively few articles concern dentistry. However, there has recently been an effective healthcare bulletin, *Dental Restoration: What Type of Filling?*, an *Effectiveness Matters* on 'Prophylactic removal of impacted third molars: is it justified?', as well as reports on systematic reviews of water fluoridation and longevity of dental restorations. Articles can be downloaded (that is, transferred to the viewer's computer) in portable document format (pdf), and these can then be viewed using widely available pdf-reader software, such as Adobe Acrobat or GhostView by GhostGum.

■ The Fédération Dentaire Internationale (FDI) has a site for National and International Guidelines and Statements, which allows the downloading (as pdf documents) of brief, multilingual recommendations on 58 dental topics, grouped into categories such as patient issues, public-health issues, dental safety, and specialized procedures.

It can be found at http://www.fdiworldental.org/resources/index.htm. The FDI site also has a 'best evidence' links page, though with a warning that the information given does not represent the official positions of the FDI World Dental Federation.

■ The Faculty of General Dental Practitioners of the Royal College of Surgeons of England offers a number of publications for sale to dentists. These give advice on practice management and contemporary, evidence based techniques, prepared by authors who are experts in their fields but who are also familiar with the constraints of general practice. The publications cannot be downloaded or read on-line, though brief details of volume content and ordering information are available (on http://www.rcseng.ac.uk/dental/fgdp/publications/). The site does, however, offer download of articles from its journal.

■ Health Evidence Bulletins – Wales is a collaborative project involving health authorities, providers of primary and secondary health care, and library and information units. It claims to act as 'a signpost to the best current evidence across a broad range of evidence types and subject areas'. Information from randomized, controlled trials is included, if available; otherwise, other high-quality evidence is sought and appraised. Printed copies of bulletins can be ordered or downloaded in pdf format from http://hebw.uwcm.ac.uk. Dental topics covered include tooth decay, periodontal diseases, cancer, joint disorders, tooth wear, and inherited anomalies.

■ The Scottish Intercollegiate Guidelines Network (SIGN) was formed in 1993, with the objective 'to improve the quality of health care for patients in Scotland by reducing variation in practice and outcome, through the development and dissemination of national clinical guidelines containing recommendations for effective practice based on current evidence. Clinical guidelines are systematically developed statements to assist practitioner and patient decisions about appropriate health care for specific clinical circumstances. Guidelines provide recommendations for effective practice in the management of clinical conditions where variations in practice are known to occur and where effective care may not be delivered uniformly throughout Scotland'.

Currently, SIGN publishes two dental clinical guidelines and quick reference guides (more are planned). These are *Preventing Dental Caries in Children at High Caries Risk: Targeted Prevention of Dental Caries in the Permanent Teeth of 6–16 Year Olds Presenting for Dental Care*[8] and *Management of Unerupted and Impacted Third Molar Teeth.*[9] These can be downloaded from http://www.sign.ac.uk/guidelines/ published/index.html in pdf format or obtained by post from Edinburgh (free within Scotland).[10] New topics may be proposed for a SIGN guideline, for which there must be evidence of variation in practice that affects patient outcomes, and a strong research base, providing evidence of effective practice.

■ A website devoted specifically to people interested in and concerned with the provision of dental primary health care is *Tuith Online*, the on-line journal of the Scottish Dental Practice Based Research Network. As well as publishing research results of interest to the providers of dental care, the site is also providing and collating guidelines for dental practitioners. The guidelines are produced under the stewardship of such organizations as SIGN, the Scottish Oral Health Group, the North West Medicines Information Centre, and others, and are listed at http://www.dundee.ac.uk/tuith/Static/info/index.htm. A high proportion of the visits to this website are to guideline pages.

■ The General Dental Council (of the UK), website http://www.gdc-uk.org, issues guidance on best practice to all registered dentists, dental hygienists, and therapists, upon first registration with the Council; any revisions are then forwarded automatically. The website, http://www.gdc-uk.org/gdcinfo.html, provides a number of advice and guidance documents (in pdf format for downloading) and details of the statutory re-certification scheme, which is being phased in over a three-year period. This scheme will help to improve patient care. Dentists who undertake continuing professional development (CPD) will become more familiar with developments in dentistry and will thereby be better placed to provide their patients with the best possible treatment.

■ The National Institute of Dental and Craniofacial Research (NIDCR), part of the National Institutes of Health in Maryland, USA, aims to promote the 'general health of the American people' by 'Knowledge acquisition through science ... and effective and efficient transfer are the means used to contribute to improved quality of health'. The NIDCR website offers a wide variety of information on oral health topics, including press releases, pamphlets, videos, reports, and guides (http://www.nidr.nih.gov/health/). Topics covered include temporomandibular disorders, amalgams, periodontal disease, oral cancer, pain, sealants, and xerostomia.

In addition to the Web-based sources of information, there are a large number of printed publications aimed at the dental team. Some of these are supported by a significant amount of advertising and contain articles which, although perhaps interesting to dental professionals, have not been subjected to the rigorous peer-review system necessary to ensure that suggested changes in practice are reliably demonstrated to be for the best. Many other publications are produced by groups which have as part of their remit the requirement to propagate research findings and suggestions for changes in practice.

For example, *APEX*, published by Leeds Medical Information at the University of Leeds, is a quarterly journal with a UK perspective, which aims to provide a forum for rapid exchange of information on aspects of general dental practice. Embracing all areas of dental practice, the aim is to help practitioners keep abreast of new developments. The quarterly bibliography includes relevant research papers, reviews, editorials, original research, and case reports, with comment on key papers selected on the basis of interest and perceived impact.

A large number of overviews, reports, and survey summaries are produced which are aimed not so much at the practitioner as at the shapers of health policy. In fact, most dentists have been found to make relatively little use of many of the sources of information available to them.[11] The problem of dissemination is the subject of Chapter 9. In the UK, general dental practitioners seem most likely to read articles from the *British Dental Journal* and *Dental Update*. There is also a great deal of confusion over what the exact meaning is of a systematic review and what the merits are.[12]

Dental Update aims to publish articles of interest to general dental practitioners. These are review or summary articles, rather than systematic reviews. An interesting development is a facility enabling dental practitioners to gain CPD points by answering questions posed on the Dental Update website at http://www.dental-update.co.uk. There is even a television channel, channel 952 (details from http://www.cpddental.tv or CPD Dental TV Ltd, High Street, Prestwood, HP16 9EU), dedicated to continuing professional development, with learning outcomes verified by the candidate's ability to answer questions and achieve a score of at least 60%.

The information available to the dental team has various levels (see Figure 8.1). However, this does not imply that evidence at lower levels is incorrect, merely that the rigour of testing, and therefore the confidence with which one can say 'This is how this should be done', are lower.

Once the evidence is presented, the next challenge is persuading clinicians to what extent they should change their established practice and adopt new ideas. The case of the prophylactic removal of pathology-free impacted third molars is one where there has been a gap between practice and recommendations. When 12 reviews were critically compared, the authors complained that sufficient details of study methods and criteria for inclusion were not supplied.[12] They concluded that there was little evidence to justify removal. *Effectiveness Matters*,[13] issued by the NHS Centre for Reviews and Dissemination in October 1998, stated that

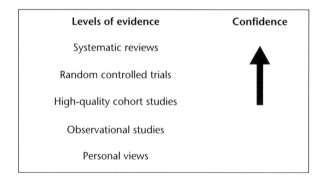

Figure 8.1 *Levels of evidence available to healthcare workers.*

third-molar surgery rates vary widely across the UK, with 35% of those prophylactically removed being disease free. This leaflet suggested that, as dentists would spend time dealing with those patients who had problems with impacted third molars rather than patients with no problems, the benefits of removal would become exaggerated. The National Institution of Clinical Evidence of the NHS in England and Wales (http://www.nice.org.uk/article.asp?a=533) recommends that healthy, impacted wisdom teeth should not be operated on because, whilst there is no evidence that this practice is of benefit to patients, there are risks accompanying surgical removal. These risks can include nerve damage, damage to other teeth, infection, bleeding, and even, rarely, death. There are also the swelling and pain in the immediate post-operative period and a financial cost to consider. Most recently, SIGN has produced a guideline, previously mentioned, *Management of Unerupted and Impacted Third Molar Teeth.*[9] The message seems to be getting through. Figure 8.2 shows that, during the 1990s, the rate of extractions was grad-

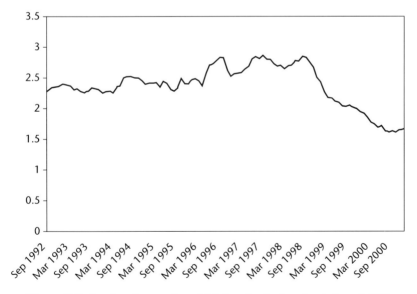

Figure 8.2 *showing the number of third molar teeth extracted per 1,000 adults attending an NHS dental examination in Scotland over an eight-year period (data courtesy of Practitioner Services Division, Edinburgh).*

ually rising in Scotland, until a sudden downturn in the popularity of this procedure in the autumn of 1998.

It is not possible to say with certainty which of the many levels of evidence led to this change of practice, but it is likely that all played a part in reinforcing the message. It is never easy to overturn an entrenched opinion, but it must be worth trying if best practice is to be maintained. As this chapter has discussed, there is an increasing range of sources that evidence may come from and of ways in which evidence and information can be and are being disseminated. The challenge for the providers of good evidence is to ensure that their voice is louder than that of those providing poor advice. The practice of evidence based dentistry is a process of life-long, problem based learning in which caring for patients should be aided by a knowledge of disease processes, prognosis, therapy, and other clinical and healthcare issues. Currently, only a minority of dental healthcare procedures fulfil the strict criteria of evidence based practice.[14] With the many sources highlighted in this chapter, the opportunities are there for dental practitioners to keep abreast of current thinking regarding what constitutes best practice, but due care must be exercised in the careful selection of sources.

'Come, pluck up heart, let's neither faint nor fear!
Better, though difficult, the right way to go,
Than wrong, though easy, where the end is woe.'[15]

References

1. Popper K, *Conjectures and refutations: the growth of scientific knowledge* (Routledge and Kegan Paul: London, 1963).
2. DHSS, *Report of the committee of enquiry into unnecessary dental treatment* (HMSO: London, 1986).
3. Richmond S, Stephens CD, Webb WG et al, Orthodontics in the general dental assessment of standards, *Br Dent J* (1993) **174**:315–329.
4. Williams AC, Bearn D, Mildinhall S et al, Cleft lip and palate care in the United Kingdom – the Clinical Standards Advisory Group (CSAG) Study. Part 2: dentofacial outcomes and patient satisfaction, *Cleft Palate Craniofac J* (2001) **38**:24–29.
5. Broder HL, Smith FB, Strauss RP, Habilitation of patients with clefts: parent

and child ratings of satisfaction with appearance and speech, *Cleft Palate Craniofac J* (1992) **29**:262–267.

6. Sackett DL and Haynes RB, On the need for evidence-based medicine, *Evidence-Based Medicine* (1995) **1**:5–6.

7. Coiera E, The Internet's challenge to health care provision, *BMJ* (1996) **31**:3–4.

8. Royal College of Physicians, Edinburgh, Preventing dental caries in children at high caries risk: targeted prevention of dental caries in the permanent teeth of 6–16 year olds presenting for dental care, *SIGN Publication Number 47* (2000).

9. Royal College of Physicians, Edinburgh, Management of unerupted and impacted third molar teeth, *SIGN Publication Number 43* (2000).

10. Scottish Intercollegiate Guidelines Network, 9 Queen Street, Edinburgh EH2 1JQ.

11. Bonner BC, Clarkson JE, McCoombes W, General dental practitioners view on the pursuit and practice of evidence-based dentistry: the results of a questionnaire, *Tuith Online*, http://www.dundee.ac.uk/tuith/Articles/rt05.htm (April 2001).

12. Song F, Landers DP, Glenny A-M et al, Prophylactic removal of impacted third molars: an assessment of published reviews, *Br Dent J* (1997) **182**:339–346.

13. NHS Centre for Reviews and Dissemination, University of York, York, UK, Prophylactic removal of third molar: is it justified? In: *Effectiveness Matters* (1998).

14. Cannavina CD, Cannavina G, Walsh TF, Effects of evidence-based treatment and consent on professional autonomy, *Br Dent J* (2000) **188**:302–306.

15. Bunyan J, *The Pilgrim's Progress* (1st Pub 1678) (Keeble NH ed, Oxford Paperbacks: Oxford, 1998).

chapter 9

Ways to disseminate and implement research evidence

Jan Clarkson, Brian C Bonner, Chris Deery and Jeremy Grimshaw

Background

Previous chapters of this book have outlined the principles and implications of the ideal of practising evidence based dentistry; the way in which evidence is accumulated, appraised and reported; and the levels of evidence made available to dental team members and others. There is a well recognized lag in the incorporation of research evidence into clinical practice. It is in fact estimated that this delay from first publication of an effective therapy until its adoption into clinical practice is over a decade. The reasons for this will be discussed in detail later in the chapter but include inertia, both personal and institutional, information overload, and difficulty in interpreting contradictory messages. Researchers and policy makers have access to a large volume of research evidence and, over the last 20 years or so, considerable progress has been made in the methods of developing clinical guidelines and in increasing their acceptance by both policy makers and clinicians.

One method of distilling research evidence into an accessible format is the use of clinical guidelines.[1-3] Clinical guidelines have been defined as 'Systematically developed statements which assist in decision making about appropriate healthcare for specific clinical conditions'.[4] However, as with any other form of evidence, the production of a guideline, no matter how well done or how eminent the body producing it, is unlikely to effect change in itself. Nonetheless, unless recommendations are incorporated into practice, the efforts of such initiatives to improve the quality of care by carrying out research will be wasted. The naïve assumption that available research evidence is routinely accessed by practitioners, appraised by them and integrated into practice, is now largely discredited. Even when knowledge of a practice guideline or a research based recommendation is acquired, it is rarely in itself sufficient to change practice. Whilst research based evidence and guidance exist, but are not incorporated into clinical practice in a timely manner, it points clearly to wasted opportunity. It is essential to seek out the most productive mechanisms by which individual and organizational change can be achieved. Thus, this chapter looks at the factors that influence the level of adoption of research evidence into dental practice: for example, implementing evidence may require health professionals to change entrenched patterns of behaviour. We are going to examine the relationship between the dissemination of research findings and their implementation, and consider some issues specific to dentistry.

An individual's beliefs, attitudes and knowledge clearly influence his or her professional behaviour; but other factors, including the practitioner's organizational, economic and community environments, will also play a part. Improvement in clinical effectiveness can only happen where there are mechanisms for change and an understanding of the change required. The complexity of changing behaviour is well recognized, and any attempt to bring about change should first involve a diagnostic analysis, an examination of potential facilitators and barriers likely to identify factors that may influence the proposed change. Choice of method of dissemination and implementation intervention should be guided by the diagnostic analysis and informed by the knowledge of relevant research.

A range of interventions has been shown to be effective in changing professional behaviour in some circumstances:

- It seems that multi-faceted interventions, targeting different barriers to change, are more likely to be effective than a single intervention.
- To succeed in effecting a change in practice, strategies need to be adequately resourced and require people armed with appropriate knowledge and skills.
- Any systematic approach to changing professional practice should include plans to monitor and evaluate, and to maintain and reinforce the changed behaviour.

Clinical governance gives all health organizations, be they government or third-party funders, the challenge of seeking quality improvements.[5–9] While 'quality' is a term which often defies precise definition in relation to health services, a key criterion is effectiveness, that is, doing more good than harm.[10] The emphasis on evidence based healthcare and the development of clinical guidelines aim to promote effectiveness and thus improve quality.[11] But this is only likely to be achieved if relevant research findings and valid guideline recommendations are appropriately incorporated into practice. In turn, this requires a change in behaviour. For example, if ways of working are shown by good research to be demonstrably less clinically effective or cost effective, they should accordingly be replaced by those shown to be more effective.

The literature on persuasive communication and advertising makes a distinction between communications that increase awareness and those that actually bring about changes in behaviour. This distinction is helpful in understanding that dissemination and implementation may be considered a spectrum of activity, where dissemination involves raising awareness of research messages and implementation involves getting the findings of research adopted into practice. The costs of implementation strategies also need to be considered. Fourteen systematic reviews that focused on interventions targeting specific behaviours were included in an *Effective Health Care Bulletin*.[12] They included interventions to improve preventive care, drug prescribing, outpatient referrals and requests for special tests. Traditionally, a simple dissemination model such as mailing published material to clinicians is used. A systematic review of the effectiveness of dissemination of written educational material (including guidelines) by publication in professional journals or mail to targeted clinicians concluded that 'the effects of printed educational materials compared with no active intervention are, at best, small across studies and of uncertain clinical significance'.[13]

The conclusion of a recent review update about the effectiveness and efficiency of guideline dissemination and implementation strategies states that 'there is an imperfect evidence base to support decisions about which guideline dissemination and implementation strategies are likely to be efficient under different circumstances. Decision makers need to use considerable judgement about how best to use the limited resources they have for guideline dissemination and implementation: to maximize population benefits based upon consideration of the potential clinical areas for clinical effectiveness activities, the likely benefits and costs required to introduce guidelines, and the likely benefits and costs as a result of any changes in provider behaviour.[14]

Multiple barriers have been identified in health services to the adoption of research findings and guidance into practice. These fall into a number of categories, such as:

- structural (financial disincentives);
- organizational (inappropriate skill mix, lack of facilities or equipment);
- peer group (local standards of care not in line with desired practice);
- individual (knowledge, attitudes, skills);
- professional/patient interaction (problems with information processing);
- patients' attitudes.

Another important factor is the 'that's the way I've always done it and I know it works' attitude.

In general dentistry, unlike in other healthcare professions, clinical competence that includes technique-sensitive procedures and materials is a consideration. However, the importance of clinical competence when considering the implementation of research evidence is unknown. At present, the general findings from healthcare research are being applied to dentistry. However, the literature rarely considers the specific barriers and confounders when trying to disseminate and implement guidelines for surgical interventions. In reality, it is normally found that considerable barriers exist to the implementation of best practice findings. Even if dissemination is carried out successfully, and primary-care dentists become aware of research findings and accept the conclusions drawn by academic and professional consensus, this often, nevertheless, does not affect an immediate change in clinical behaviour. This presents something of a dilemma of how best to address barriers that exist at other levels.

Research into the dissemination and implementation of research findings has generally been conducted in medicine. Although many of the barriers to, and promoters of, professional change discussed in the rest of this chapter may be similar in both medicine and dentistry, it cannot be taken for granted that what applies to one applies to the other. Similarly, the effect of implementation strategies may also differ between professions.

Dentistry itself is not uniform and there are, for example, likely to be differences in the effectiveness of approaches in primary dental care compared to secondary care. Returning to the comparison between dentistry and medicine, it may well be that secondary dental care and medical care have many similarities, but it is likely that primary medical care and dental care may differ markedly. One reason for this belief is the differing funding systems within which these groups work. For example, in the United Kingdom, general medical practitioners work principally within a capitation scheme, whereas general dental practitioners work mainly under a fee-for-item system.

McGlone et al reviewed the challenges to changing behaviour in dentistry.[15] They recognized that our knowledge in this field is somewhat limited. Factors they identified as being specific barriers to change in dentistry included (see categories identified above):

■ profession's perception of patients (structural);

- patients' attitudes to dental health and the cost of dental care[16] (structural);
- fear of medico-legal action[17] (structural/individual);
- treatment-funding system (structural barrier);
- time lost to practice when attending courses (structural/organizational);

With regard to facilitators of change in dentistry:

- Knowledge of a practice and attendance at continuing education courses have been shown to promote the adoption of a new practice. For example, knowledge about the appropriate use of pit and fissure sealants has been shown to correlate with their use.[18] However, educational interventions tend to have broad rather than specific effects on behaviour.
- The same study also suggested that the use of professionals complementary to dentistry also promoted the use of sealants. Although an interesting finding in itself, why does having a hygienist in your practice result in your placing more sealants? Is it that the use of a hygienist makes the adoption of a procedure more cost effective, or is it that practitioners who employ hygienists are early adopters? Further work is required to explore these issues, as there appears to be a correlation between some factors without there being an understanding of why this is the case.

In dentistry there has been some research into the effectiveness of differing strategies to promote adherence to guidelines. Unfortunately, this has not yielded particularly promising results.

A randomized, controlled trial using the appropriateness of referral as the outcome measure demonstrated that guidelines for orthodontic referrals did not influence the behaviour of general dental practitioners.[19] Two methods of dissemination were planned: guidelines sent to practices, with both questionnaires and a re-issue after six months, and a series of seminars as follow-up. In reality, although the guidelines were well received, there was no take-up of the seminars, which were cancelled. On the basis of analysis of the data collected, it was concluded that even when referral guidelines were produced using optimum methods, and disseminated using the only pragmatic methods available, they did not have an effect.

Another randomized, controlled trial has evaluated the implementation of guidelines for the appropriate management of third molar teeth using a multifaceted approach.[20] The strategies used in this study were: 1) passive dissemination, 2) audit and feedback, 3) computer-aided learning, and 4) a combination of all three strategies. Again, this study was unable to detect any difference in the effectiveness of the strategies. Another study reported that the interventions did have an influence on practitioner knowledge and intention.[21]

We are at a time of great change in dental education in the United Kingdom, with the introduction of mandatory continuing professional development. It is to be hoped that this will encourage reflective professionalism. The test of this will be whether, in five to ten years' time, dental practice is demonstrably more evidence based.

There is a need for considerable research into dentistry, drawing on the experiences from medicine to identify the most effective strategies to disseminate and implement research findings and thus promote best practice and ensure the best outcome for patients.

Dissemination

It is possible that passive dissemination of evidence serves as an important function in increasing awareness of the most effective treatments and interventions. The provision of summaries of research conclusions and carefully formulated practice guidelines might lead to tangible changes in dental practice. However, at the present time we do not have evidence of how best to present this for dental professionals and patients. Studies need to be conducted comparing different ways of presenting summaries of judgements about the quality of evidence and the balance between benefits, harms and costs. The patient attending for dental treatment also needs assurance regarding the basis and quality of care received. The best method of communicating this is yet to be established.

The aim of dissemination is to raise awareness of research evidence. To this end various mechanisms exist, none of which can achieve such consciousness raising in isolation. Dissemination methods range from word-of-mouth from peer groups or from specialists consulted in specific cases, through the many guideline documents and sheets made available or mailed directly to practices, to information picked up from reading journals and the specialist press. There is no doubt that the amount of published information available is prodigious. Too much information can be even more of a problem than too little. This overload causes problems for the dental professional, trying to identify relevant information, and for the information disseminator competing for the attention of the target audience. The case for improvements in practice must be more persuasive than any harmful advice, incorrect recommendations or folklore.

Encouragement to keep up to date with new ideas and modern practice comes from professional colleagues, patients, dental assurance schemes, dental professional organizations and associations, the government, and the individual's desire not to be performing less than his/her best. It would be hoped that newly qualified dental professionals would be up to date with current practice, but for this to be true, the people responsible for their training should be up to date and trained to disseminate evidence effectively.

One important problem area is the gap between the academic paper, which is unlikely to come to the attention of a busy dental worker, and the practice-friendly, quick-reference guide or article in a professional journal. Academic papers are often published in respected but esoteric journals to satisfy research assessment exercises, grant-awarding bodies, or to bolster curricula vitae to aid in career progression. Not all authors may consider it their responsibility also to publish in a more accessible format, or may be unaware that there is a problem. This is where systematic review bodies such as The Cochrane Collaboration come into their own. They undertake to scan academic literature and ensure that relevant and practice-enhancing improvements are restated in a more practitioner-friendly format. Communication skills are vital in getting the message across to members of the dental team from researchers, but also in the interaction between the dental team and the patient. The mass media also play a role in dissemination, both to the practitioner and the patient. It is becoming increasingly common for patients to search and find evidence themselves; having done this, they then question their carer, asking about the availability and appropriateness of treatment. Unfortunately, the quality of the information is very variable.

Implementation

Traditionally, the dissemination of research evidence is where efforts to change practice have stopped. More recently, the need to actively promote the uptake of research knowledge has been identified. A number of different implementation strategies are available, for example audit and feedback, educational outreach visits, reminders; and there is increasing interest at policy levels in the use of more active implementation strategies. However, our knowledge about their effectiveness in different settings remains limited. More often, the choice of strategy is based on familiarity, rather than scientific evidence that it will make a difference.[22] Research effort in evidence based dentistry needs to be complemented by research into how best to implement this evidence into general and specialist practice.

In order for implementation to be effective, not only do the processes of dissemination and implementation need to be effective and efficient, but sufficient and adequate resources need to be available to provide the most effective interventions, as well as a supportive culture to make changes in routine practice. The bottom line is that it is not those involved in developing the summaries of best evidence who need information of effective implementation strategies, but those responsible for the quality of care within provider organizations.

A wide range of research methods has been used to investigate the effectiveness of different strategies for getting research evidence into practice. These include before-and-after studies, time-series studies and randomized, controlled trials. The best source of a decision about the choice of implementation strategies comes from systematic reviews. Unfortunately, at present, there are very few trials of methods to disseminate and implement research findings in dentistry, making systematic reviews impossible. Therefore, at the moment, dentistry has to look to other branches of the medical literature to identify effective methods.

As described in previous chapters, systematic reviews of rigorous evaluations of implementation interventions increase the precision of findings by combining results from different studies. They can also explore the consistency of findings between studies and investigate the generalizability of findings across different settings, professional groups and behaviours. High-quality systematic reviews have been conducted, but do not include a single study from dentistry.

The Cochrane Effective Practice and Organisation of Care review group (EPOC) aims to undertake systematic reviews of interventions to improve the quality of care. EPOC reviewers have conducted an overview of previously conducted systematic reviews of provider behaviour change, summarizing the current state of knowledge.[23]

Fifty-one reviews published up to the end of 1998 were identified and included. The implementation strategies that had been considered could be divided into three broad categories: strategies that are ineffective in most studies; strategies that are effective in some studies but not in others; and strategies effective in most studies. Largely ineffective strategies are passive dissemination and didactic educational sessions, in which information is presented to a passive audience. These strategies may raise awareness of an issue, but they have little or no impact on practice. Strategies that vary in their effectiveness are audit and feedback, local consensus conferences, opinion leaders and patient-mediated interventions. These may be effective in some circumstances, but it is not yet clear which circumstances these are. The audit process seeks to improve patient care and outcomes through systematic review of care against explicit criteria. Where indicated, changes are implemented at an individual, team or service level, and further monitoring is used to confirm improvement in healthcare delivery.

This overview of systematic reviews suggests that a variety of implementation strategies have the potential to be effective under certain conditions. However, the evidence is sparse for many interventions, and the reviews themselves are of variable quality with common methodological flaws.

High-quality clinical guidelines have multiple applications in practice.[24] These include their primary role of allowing clinicians to identify the most effective treatments and healthcare interventions rapidly, but also to assist in the presentation of evidence for standards in audit and as a source of educational material. Whereas guideline development is most efficiently undertaken at national or international level, guideline implementation, in contrast, is largely a local activity. The recognition that passive dissemination of guidelines is not enough to improve the quality of healthcare leads to a greater emphasis on active implementation strategies. These are undertaken at the local level, with the strategy selected according to evidence about its effectiveness. The extent to which evidence base is used when planning local implementation activities is uncertain. Owing to the greater availability of resources, guidelines developed at a national or international level are more likely to lead to more valid conclusions than locally developed guidelines, although this has never been tested.[25] However, there is a tension here, as the extent of implementation of guidelines at the local level is greater if those applying the guideline have a sense of ownership, which is more likely to be the case the more closely to the local level the guidelines are developed.

The costs of a dissemination and implementation strategy and the consequential costs of care need to be considered.

Evidence of the effectiveness of implementation is not always readily available. One strategy is to consult reviews of interventions in which the main outcome considered was the change in performance. In one such study, it was concluded that the authors of few reviews attempted to explicitly link findings to theories of behavioural change.[26] Multifaceted interventions and interactive educational meetings were found to be the most effective at promoting behavioural change, with audit, local opinion leaders, and local consensus processes having variable effectiveness. Educational materials and lectures were found to have little or no effect.

The importance of considering theoretical models of behaviour change to inform the development and implementation of interventions intended to change behaviour is not generally recognized. There is little in the dental literature to support the adoption of specific models or approaches. Although it is possible to acknowledge the generalizability of these to dentistry, more research is required to guide decision-making. Learning theory can be used to promote change by modifying factors that control behaviour. Behaviour in a particular way tends to increase if followed by positive reinforcement consequences, such as educational credits or finance. The effectiveness depends on how desirable the reinforcement consequence is. Similarly, negative behaviour followed by removal of a desired consequence is likely to decrease undesirable behaviour. Social cognition models, instead of changing the individual's environment, influence factors such as beliefs, attitudes and intentions. Beliefs that are considered important are perceived benefits, weighed against barriers such as costs, perceptions about the attitudes of important others to the behaviour, and the belief in one's ability to perform a particular behaviour. Theoretically, using planned interventions, the sequence of stages that individuals go through (for example to adopt evidence based healthcare) can be negotiated in sequence and change secured. However, evidence would suggest that it is important to target specific groups and work closely with them to discover their needs, barriers and drivers for change, rather than adopting blanket policies.[27] Models of organizational change emphasize the complex nature of the environment that we work in and acknowledge the requirement to change internal and external influencing factors.

Summary

The reasons research evidence is not routinely adopted into practice are complex, and for dentistry we have very little reliable information on this topic. We know from medical practice that information problems are critical, with ineffective communication and uncertainty in the validity of the research evidence being important. In addition, where evidence based guidelines derived from research are at odds with an individual patient's preference, the individual's wishes tend to take precedence.

The effect of stress has been recognized as a barrier to behaviour change for individuals and teams. Ignoring the difficulties within the job or expecting change with fewer resources will create additional stress and can lead to resentment which, in turn, may fuel resistance. Without motivation, maintenance of the status quo and the 'this is the way I've always done it' attitude may prevail.

This chapter has outlined some of the difficulties associated with the dissemination and implementation of research evidence and the adoption of evidence based practice. It should not be forgotten that successful change is unlikely to happen unless the people with the necessary skills and knowledge exist to lead and apply the dissemination and implementation activities. Strategies must include mechanisms to monitor and evaluate the success of attempts to alter practice and behaviour and plans to reinforce and maintain the message.

Nevertheless, it is clear that there are 'no magic bullets' when it comes to choosing implementation strategies.[28] Interventions based on a prior assessment of potential barriers to change may be more effective, and multifaceted interventions targeting different barriers to change are more likely to be effective than single interventions, but they are also likely to be more costly.

There is a substantial body of rigorous evidence that can be used to inform decisions about implementation strategies. This needs to be used alongside other types of knowledge and activity to maximize the likelihood of improving dental healthcare and management and moving towards the best available practice.

References

1. Faculty of General Dental Practitioners (UK), *Clinical examination and record-keeping. Good practice guidelines* (The Royal College of Surgeons of England: London, UK).
2. SIGN Publication Number 47 (2000), *Preventing dental caries in children at high*

caries risk: Targeted prevention of dental caries in the permanent teeth of 6–16 year olds presenting for dental care (Royal College of Physicians: Edinburgh).

3. SIGN Publication Number 43 (2000), *Management of unerupted and impacted third molar teeth* (Royal College of Physicians: Edinburgh).

4. Institute of Medicine Committee on Clinical Practice Guidelines, *Guidelines for clinical practice: from development to use* (National Academy Press: Washington, DC, 1992).

5. Department of Health, *The new NHS: modern dependable*, UK White Paper (The Stationery Office: London, 1997).

6. Scottish Office, *Designed to care: renewing the NHS in Scotland* (Stationery Office: Edinburgh, 1997).

7. Welsh Office, *NHS Wales: putting patients first* (Stationery Office: London, 1998).

8. Secretary of State for Health, *A first class service: quality in the new NHS* (Stationery Office: London, 1997).

9. Scally G, Donaldson L, Clinical governance and the drive for quality improvement in the new NHS in England, *BMJ* (1998) **317**:61–65.

10. Maxwell R, Perspectives in NHS Management, *BMJ* (1984) **288**:1470–1472.

11. Agency for Health Care Policy and Research, *Using clinical guidelines to evaluate quality of care*, Volume 1: Issues. (US Dept of Health and Human Services, Public Health Service, 1995) (AHCPR Pub. No. 95-0045).

12. NHS Centre for Reviews and Dissemination, Getting evidence into practice, *Effective Health Care Bulletin* (1999) **5**:1–16. www.york.ac.uk/inst/crd/ehc51.pdf

13. Grimshaw JM, Shirran L, Thomas RE et al, Changing provider behaviour: an overview of systematic reviews of interventions, *Med Care* (2001) **39**:II-2–II-45.

14. Grimshaw JM, Thomas RE, Maclennan G et al, Effectiveness and efficiency of guideline dissemination and implementation strategies. *Health Technol Assess* (submitted for publication 2002).

15. McGlone P, Watt R, Sheiham A, Evidence-based dentistry: an overview of the challenges in changing professional practice, *BDJ* (2001) **190**:636–639.

16. Kay EJ, Blinkhorn AS, A qualitative investigation of factors governing dentists' treatment philosophies, *BDJ* (1996) **180**:171–176.

17. Rushton VE, Horner K, Worthington HV, Factors influencing frequency of bitewing radiography in general dental practice, *Commun Dentistry Oral Epidemiol* (1996) **24**:272–276.

18. Main PA, Lewis DW, Hawkins RJ, A survey of general dentists in Ontario, Part 1 sealant usage and knowledge, *J Canad Dent Assoc* (1997) **63**:543–553.

19. O'Brien K, Wright J, Conboy F et al, The effect of orthodontic referral guidelines: a randomised controlled trial, *BDJ* (2000) **188**:392–397.

20. Bahrami M, Bonetti D, Clarkson JE et al, Effectiveness of different dissemination and implementation strategies for evidence based guidelines for third molar problems in primary dental care, *7th European Forum on Quality Improvement in Health Care*, 2002.

21. Bonetti D, Johnston M, Pitts NB et al, Can implementation intention interventions be used to eliminate a behaviour? *Proceedings from the European Health Psychology Society Annual Conference*, 2001.

22. Grol R, Beliefs and evidence in changing clinical practice, *BMJ* (1997) **315**:418–421.
23. Mowatt G, Grimshaw JM, Davis D et al, Getting Evidence into practice – the work of the Cochrane Effective Practice and Organisation of Care Group (EPOC), *J Contin Educ Health Prof* (2001) **21**:55–60.
24. Clarkson JE, Grimshaw JM, *Community Dental Health* (2000) **17**:1–2.
25. Cluzeau F, Littlejohns P, Grimshaw JM et al, Development of a generic methodology for appraising the quality of clinical guidelines, *Int J Qual Health Care* (1999) **11**:21–28.
26. Bero LA, Grilli R, Grimshaw JM et al, Closing the gap between research and practice: an overview of systematic reviews of interventions to promote implementation of research findings by health care professionals, *BMJ* (1998) **317**:465–468.
27. Firth-Cozens J, Health promotion: changing behaviour towards evidence-based health care, *Int J Qual Health Care* (1997) **6**:205–211.
28. Oxman AD, Thomson MA, Davis DA et al, No magic bullets: a systematic review of 102 trials of interventions to improve professional practice, *CMAJ* (1995) **153**:1423–1431.

chapter 10

What effect will evidence based dentistry have on clinical practice?

Bob Ireland and Jayne E Harrison

In the context of clinical practice, evidence based dentistry is defined as the conscientious, explicit and judicious use of current best evidence in making decisions about the care of individual patients. Or more simply, trying to ensure that general dental practitioners get the results of good up-to-date research applied to their own practice as quickly as possible.[1] Questions are now frequently being asked as to why we should adopt evidence based dentistry in clinical dental practice and if we do, what effect it will have. Understandably, we are always reluctant to change the way we do things unless there is a good reason for doing so. Therefore these questions need to be given careful consideration, because the adoption of an evidence based approach to clinical practice will result in profound changes to the way we think and work in the future. It will also impact on every member of the dental team.

Why introduce evidence based dentistry into clinical practice?

The purchasers of health care are, in many ways, no different from any consumer who purchases a product. For example, someone buying an electric razor would expect it to carry out the function for which it was designed and would expect it to work well for what is, in their opinion, a reasonable period of time. At the time of purchase, they will have the opportunity to compare it with similar products or to obtain comparative information from independent organizations, such as the Consumers Association (UK), which assess quality and value for money. Having bought the product, if it fails to perform according to their expectations, they will more than likely return to the supplier for an explanation and remedial action. Patients attending primary dental care clinics are no different from other consumers and they are starting to judge, in a similar way, the quality of the dental care they receive.

We generally think that the purchasers of health care are members of the general public, that is, our patients. However, purchasers fall into a number of different groups as, by definition, purchasers are those who are paying for our service. In the UK, the National Health Service (NHS) is the largest single purchaser of primary dental health care. Like all national healthcare systems, it is constrained by limited resources. It is therefore very keen to get the best quality healthcare provision for minimum financial outlay. Many countries have other organizations concerned with the funding of primary dental health care such as insurance companies, corporate bodies etc. The question all these purchasers have in common and on which their attention is focused, is whether they are getting value for money. They are all starting to demand the evidence to indicate the quality of the dental health care delivered; both in terms of how it is delivered and the outcome of any treatment intervention or advice that is given. In essence, the purchasers are asking 'Does the treatment work?', 'Is it likely to produce the most successful outcome?', 'How do we know it works?'. Funding agencies (be they public or private) may withdraw funding from ineffective or unnecessary treatments such as the removal of asymptomatic third molars, or conversely, may start funding interventions that have been shown to be effective but have previously been unavailable, such as nicotine replacement therapy. However, patients may have other priorities and decide to fund alternative treatments that fulfil their personal requirements. For example, a cosmetic need may override financial or clinical effectiveness requirements.

It will not be sufficient for us as practitioners to respond by basing our evidence of success or failure on a few personal experiences or word of mouth from colleagues. Consumers are becoming much more powerful in demanding quality and we will have an obligation to respond. With the development of new information sources and technologies, patients will, in future, have ready access to a vast amount of clinical information, much of it obtained from the Internet and electronic databases.[2] This will make patients very much more informed and aware of what is available in the way of treatment alternatives and what is meant by evidence based dentistry. But are patients better informed or misinformed? Unfortunately at the present time, much of the information that is available on the Internet is of questionable value and can be both inaccurate or misleading since there is no quality control or peer review. The information could have come from a recognized international expert or from a crank. Information often originates from personal opinion or from commercial companies who have a vested interest in promoting their own products. Therefore, there is a need to develop some means of assuring the quality of this information so that patients are not misinformed. For this reason it is important for us to be able to counter such material with accurate evidence from valid studies. These consumer demands cannot be ignored since they have the potential to be a very powerful driving force for the introduction of evidence based dentistry. We, as practitioners, will need to be proactive, rather than reactive, in meeting this challenge if we are to continue to provide an effective and worthwhile service for our patients.

What can be influenced by the evidence based approach?

The answer to this is 'almost anything!' The areas can however, be grouped into the three broad categories of structures, processes and outcomes.

The structures relate to the equipment we use within our practices. These include handpieces, autoclaves, fibre-optic lights and clinical cameras to name but a few. They can all be evaluated to determine their function, reliability and cost-effectiveness.

Processes are the methods that we use to undertake a procedure so that we achieve the best outcome efficiently, safely and cost-effectively. These methods are usually guided by either written or verbal protocols and where appropriate, can be utilized by any member of the dental team.

Both structures and processes will have an influence on the clinical outcome. Measuring outcomes forms the basis of the evidence based approach. Most of the activity in clinical practice is aimed at the treatment and prevention of caries and periodontal disease. In looking at outcomes, it is important to establish whether the treatment is effective in achieving this and whether having given preventive advice it results in an attitude change on the part of the patient and the consequent reduction of the level of disease.

What is the process of undertaking evidence based dentistry in clinical practice?

Initially this can seem pretty daunting, but if a systematic and logical approach is adopted it is well within the scope and ability of any practitioner. The process adopts a sequence of stages which it is important to follow. These are outlined in Figure 10.1.

Define your problem

This is most important, because it is easy to be confused or unclear about what the real clinical question is. Confusion at the start can result in much wasted time looking for the wrong evidence and frequently results in an inappropriate or irrelevant answer.

Search for the evidence

A useful starting point for the busy practitioner can be the Internet. There are plenty of websites available and helpful starting places are the Evidence Based Dentistry or Cochrane Oral Health Group websites.[3,4] The process of searching for the evidence has been covered in Chapter 2 of this book. However, it is worth remembering that, when searching electronic databases, such as MEDLINE, you will only identify about 50% of the research information on any given topic.

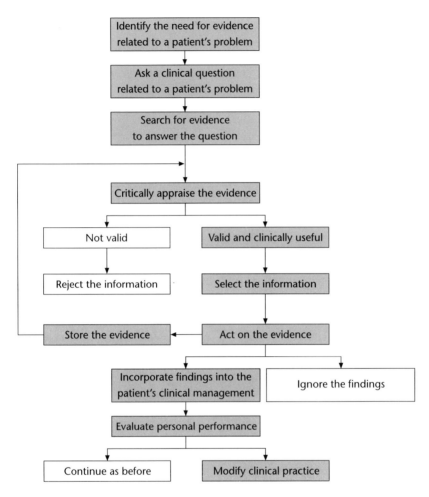

Figure 10.1 *Process of evidence based care.*

Critically appraise the evidence

When the evidence is located, it should be both the best and the latest. Evidence is constantly being updated and it is easy to accept evidence from an early paper which has since been superseded by studies which have refuted earlier conclusions. The evidence must, therefore, be critically appraised to establish whether the conclusions stated are valid.

Poor evidence should be rejected. Unfortunately, the critical appraisal of the literature requires the acquisition and development of skills. These are readily learnt and by asking a few key questions, the busy practitioner can start to identify relevant studies from those that will add little to his or her knowledge base. The basis of critical appraisal has been covered in Chapter 3 of this book and further details of this process can be obtained from other publications.[5,6] There are also a number of courses which will enable practitioners to become skilled in this important area.[3,7] It is not sufficient to assume that, just because a study is published, a definitive answer has been provided. For example, a recent study showed there to be a direct link between the measles, mumps and rubella (MMR) vaccine and the incidence of autism.[8] This had a significant negative effect on the uptake of vaccination in young children. However, other studies, including a much larger one carried out in Finland,[9] have not shown an association between the vaccine and autism. This highlights the need to refer to and appraise new evidence and illustrates the reason why systematic reviews of the literature can give a better overall picture of the evidence than single studies especially where the results of studies are variable.

Is the evidence valid and relevant?

Having appraised the evidence it is necessary to decide whether it is valid and relevant. Does the evidence apply to your particular clinical situation and does it apply to your patient? If it is not valid then it can be rejected and you can continue as before. However, if it is valid and clinically useful then the findings can be incorporated into the clinical management of the patient and will hopefully result in a beneficial change in your usual clinical practice procedures.

Evaluate personal performance

Having introduced a change to clinical practice you need to know whether the intended beneficial change does actually take place and the clinical outcome is improved. This process of analysis can be quick to achieve, for example, if you were analyzing the result of changing your technique with respect to the delivery of regional block anaesthesia.

However, other changes, such as the effect of a technique change on the longevity of posterior composite restorations, may not be measurable for several years and therefore take considerably longer to evaluate.

Store the evidence
It should be possible for you to efficiently access the evidence on which you acted so that it can be referred to on a future occasion. This is now much easier with the advent of electronic filing and data storage systems. It is however, still useful to retain paper-based copies of research papers for additional backup.

Update your evidence
It is easy to forget that new evidence is constantly becoming available and may contradict previous research. The basis for clinical practice should be a process of continuous review. Clinical questions should therefore be revisited on a regular basis and new evidence appraised, rejected or accepted, applied and stored.

What is the difference between evidence based dentistry and clinical experience?

Evidence based dentistry attempts to answer clinical questions based on a critical review of the best available scientific evidence, clinical experience and scientific knowledge.[10] It is necessary to maintain a balance between these three sources of knowledge in order to achieve the best outcomes. When the concept of evidence based medicine (EBM) was first coined clinicians were worried that clinical practice would become 'cookbook' medicine. However, the advocates of evidence based practice acknowledge the fact that good clinicians use both individual clinical expertise together with the best available evidence and that neither alone is enough. Without clinical expertise practice risks becoming dominated by 'evidence', which, although excellent as a generalization, may be inapplicable or inappropriate for an individual patient. Conversely, without the current best evidence, clinical practice may be based more on anecdote or tradition and risks becoming rapidly out of date which surely is not in the best interests of our patients. The best evidence can inform, but can never replace individual clinical expertise because it is this expertise which decides whether the evidence applies to the individual patient and, if so, how it should be integrated into a clinical decision. The practice of EBM has therefore evolved to mean the integration of individual clinical expertise with the best available evidence from systematic research.[11] The contribution that clinical experience makes to successful outcomes is important. This is true in arriving at the correct diagnosis, treatment plan and the skill with which the treatment is delivered. However, there is a great tendency for practitioners to be excessively influenced by a recent treatment success or failure on an individual patient without considering it in the context of a wider experience or in the light of a review of further research evidence. If we are not careful, clinical experience can be a process of repeating the same mistake many times over many years. Research evidence will usually be based on studies of large numbers of patients or interventions and will therefore give a much more accurate reflection of what is happening. This should be used as an adjunct to sound clinical judgement.

How do we get evidence based research into primary dental care?

Audit might be described as the first stage in developing the research process. Audit is the process of identifying and monitoring a process or outcome, comparing this with a previously and externally defined 'gold standard', modifying the process to try to achieve the gold standard and then re-monitoring to see whether the changes have achieved the desired result. The process is described as a cycle, or more correctly as a spiral, since it is necessary to continue to review the standard against which the process is benchmarked, and standards are not static. The result should be to gradually improve quality of care. Those dentists practising within the National Health Service in the UK are now required to undertake clinical audit as part of their terms of service. A logical progression from clinical audit is to embark upon a more in-depth research study based on problems encountered in routine clinical practice. This, however, requires either the acquisition of additional research skills or collaboration with academic researchers or both.

There is a tendency, however, for the practitioner to practice in isolation from clinical researchers. Frequently, we, as primary care practitioners, think that researchers don't appreciate the real world of clinical practice. Researchers, on the other hand, can often feel frustrated that research is not carried through and applied to clinical practice and that practitioners continue to treat patients using outmoded philosophies, techniques or materials, which fail to take account of the evidence generated by more recent research. As practitioners we can find it difficult to change our way of operating to adopt new techniques and concepts. There is a need to bring both practitioners and researchers together to work as a partnership in linking the research evidence with the clinical application. This collaboration can only be mutually beneficial in appreciating the contribution that the two groups can make so this relationship can be seen as symbiotic. For this reason the practitioner should grasp the opportunity to promote and fully participate in evidence based research in the primary care setting. After all, practitioners are ideally placed to determine the relevant areas of research with respect to patients' needs based on clinical experience and then to apply the results of that research in everyday clinical practice. Primary care research provides an opportunity to develop collaboration with academic units. Research is very much a team exercise and requires the amalgamation of a number of different skills. Not only is the practitioner a key player in such a team but participation allows the development of new skills which can be a useful asset in evaluating clinical care provision. Carrying out research provides a better understanding of the process of establishing the quality of a material or piece of equipment from an evidence based standpoint. Participating in research not only provides the practitioner with a sense of involvement, which is more likely to lead to changes in clinical practice, but also enables the practitioner to better evaluate and critically appraise published research reports. In developing this partnership the practitioner should not be regarded as simply a data gatherer to provide research material for another academically led clinical study but as an equal contributor and beneficiary.

The practitioner also has the unique opportunity to utilize a vast patient database of clinical information which is invaluable in analyzing and evaluating the effects of clinical intervention and the outcomes achieved. The practitioner is in the ideal position to identify the main problems of clinical practice and therefore can provide a valuable lead as to the important areas of research. This can be achieved by retrospective or prospective evaluation of individual patients or selected patient groups. It also provides an opportunity for practitioners in different practice locations to get together and collaborate on research by aggregating data from each of their practices thereby widening the evidence base available. However, evidence derived from analysis of computerized databases is quite low down the scale of the hierarchy of evidence (Figure 10.2)[12,13] and as such, by itself, is not particularly valid. Investigating these problems can stimulate enthusiasm on the part of the practitioner, which can significantly improve professional satisfaction and make a challenging and beneficial contribution to the activity of routine clinical practice.

Practitioners frequently rely on the assertions made by materials' manufacturers as to the quality of their products. These assertions may

---

Anecdotal case report
Cross-sectional   survey
Case series without a control
Case–control observational study
Cohort study with a literature control
Analyses using computer databases
Cohort study with a historical control group
Unconfirmed randomized controlled clinical trial
Confirmed definitive randomized controlled clinical trials
Systematic review of randomized controlled clinical trials

Figure 10.2 *Hierarchy of evidence.*

be true but it is often the case that evidence from routine clinical practice has not contributed to the claims made by the manufacturers and
their quality may only be based on in vitro studies or clinical studies
under highly controlled conditions. In addition, the information made
available by manufacturers may be very selective. After all, they are
unlikely to publicize the properties of a material that compare less
favourably with those of their competitors. The important question is
how a product behaves in the real world of general dental practice rather
than in the laboratory or the hands of the specialist who is not necessarily subjected to the time and cost constraints of general practice.

How can evidence based research influence clinical practice?

Much of what we do is not based on sound evidence. Studies in the US
have estimated that less than half of the health care provided is evidence based.[14] It is worthwhile looking at a few examples of the influence
of evidence based research on decision making in routine clinical
practice.

The issue of whether impacted asymptomatic wisdom teeth should be
prophylactically removed has been the subject of debate for some time.
The NHS Centre for Reviews and Dissemination, at the University of
York, undertook a study of 12 objectively selected reviews and concluded that, in the absence of good evidence to support prophylactic
removal, there appears to be no justification for the removal of pathology-free impacted third molars. This has resulted in a guideline for
current good clinical practice and has been endorsed by the National
Institute for Clinical Excellence (NICE).[15] The Scottish Intercollegiate
Guideline Network (SIGN)[16] has also produced a guideline following a
systematic review,[17] but because of the absence of reliable long-term
research evidence for both reviews, they need to be supported by clinical
trials.

In assessing a surgical technique for the removal of lower third
molars, Robinson and Smith carried out a randomized controlled trial in

a UK dental school. They concluded that the conventional UK method of lingual retraction using a Howarth's retractor, to protect the lingual nerve, is invalid and lingual retraction should be avoided to reduce the risk of lingual nerve damage.[18]

Scurria et al[19] undertook a systematic review on the survival rate of fixed bridges. They concluded that that only 15% were removed or in need of replacement 10 years after insertion. This provides a useful benchmark against which a practitioner could measure his or her own performance.

Who funds evidence based research?

Carrying out any kind of research in practice involves a not inconsiderable time commitment and therefore frequently raises the question of who will pay for it? Fortunately, major funding sources are beginning to acknowledge the important contribution of primary care research. For example, the NHS has recently invested £5 million in a national primary dental care research and development programme.[20] The NHS is actively supporting the development of a research capability within primary care teams.[21,22] Funding opportunities are also available from the Faculty of General Dental Practitioners,[23] the British Dental Association[24] (e.g. Shirley Glasstone Hughes Awards) and from commercial companies.

How can technological development help?

The transfer of technology from the research environment to clinical practice is not easy. Information technology (IT) applications in dentistry are at last beginning to provide the tools necessary to realistically implement the retrospective evaluation of clinical activity and the effect that treatment intervention has on a patient's oral health. Until recently, most dentists have recorded all clinical patient data on paper-based record card systems. This may be very safe and reliable but has the great disadvantage that accessing and collating data for analysis is a long and tedious process. For this reason it is rarely, if ever, undertaken. This is very disappointing since this data probably could provide pointers to relevant clinical questions. Computers allow the storage of clinical data in an electronic format. The potential is there to retrieve this data almost instantaneously and with the loss of little or no additional clinical time. The manufacturers of clinical software systems need to be encouraged to develop their systems so that reporting functions can be undertaken quickly and efficiently. This would allow the practitioner to evaluate the effect of intervention or advice on the oral health of a single patient or group of patients. Not only could this be carried out on an individual dentist basis, but the data could also be compared with that of colleagues in similar practising situations. It would also provide the opportunity to measure performance or outcomes against pre-defined goals. This is the basis of self-audit or self-evaluation. These goals or standards can be guided by the results of evidence based research.

Supra-national bodies, such as the World Health Organization, already collate considerable amounts of data relating to healthcare issues and make it freely available by means of databases accessible via the Internet.[25,26] The development of software systems will allow clinicians to record all clinical data without, hopefully, having to be computer experts. The capture of the clinical data should not be an additional burden since it is already part of good clinical practice. There should be no additional time commitment, which might take the practitioner away from clinical activity, since the economic pressures of the busy general practice are important when adopting this new technology. Unfortunately software manufacturers haven't fully appreciated the enormous potential for self-analysis that their systems might provide. This is largely because practitioners have not demanded such a function. With the increasing emphasis on clinical governance this facility is likely to become of increasing importance in the future. It is up to dentists and the other members of the dental team to demand this audit function when reviewing the purchase of IT systems. It must be remembered however, that the validity and reliability of this data may be questionable and should therefore be interpreted with caution.

Clinical dental software systems provide the additional opportunity to integrate decision support and expert systems into the electronic patient record. It is extremely difficult for the busy practitioner to keep up to date with the latest techniques and in a busy practice, important questions for the patient when trying to arrive at a diagnosis may be forgotten or over-looked. Decision support systems provide guidance for the practitioner, based on the latest available evidence, on the most appropriate way to manage a clinical problem. Expert systems combine a knowledge base and an inference mechanism to lead a dentist to arrive at either a diagnosis or the most appropriate treatment pathway. These systems should be developed from evidence based research. It is likely that, in the future, practitioners will come to be increasingly reliant on these support systems since failure to adopt appropriate evidence based clinical practice may result, at best, in poor outcomes and at worst, in litigation by patients.

Who should be involved?

There are opportunities for all members of the dental team to participate in evidence based dentistry. Hygienists spend a considerable amount of time providing patient education and undertaking clinical interventions and then monitoring the outcomes on an individual basis. However, there is plenty of evidence to suggest that patients can become more knowledgeable about oral health, but little or no evidence to suggest that the knowledge gained results in a positive behaviour change.[27] It is also important that a hygienist should know whether the treatment that is being undertaken is based on evidence. These important research areas remain to be investigated to justify the investment in both time and money by the patients and there is no reason to suggest that hygienists shouldn't participate fully in this research. Dental therapists are involved in simple restorative procedures and therefore are very aware of the problems encountered in utilizing new materials. They have the opportunity to participate with the other members of the dental team in initiating and participating in research that will help to address many relevant research issues.

Dental nurses play an increasingly important role in the maintenance of infection control. This is now an important and significant part of clinical practice. Dental nurses need to be aware of the contribution they are making and the evidence base on which infection control procedures and policies are based. Nurses in general medical practices are frequently adopting the role of research team leader and there is no reason why dental nurses in general dental practice shouldn't follow their example.

There are opportunities for other non-clinical members of the dental team, such as receptionists and practice managers, to be involved in research to evaluate and improve the process of healthcare delivery. For example, they have the opportunity to sample patient opinion by means of questionnaires or surveys which will provide valuable information on both the clinical and non-clinical aspects of a practice.

Summary

The incorporation of an evidence based approach to clinical practice has the potential to affect many aspects of our working lives. It has the potential to alter the way we think about clinical problems, the way we collect and process clinical data and may change our prescribing due to shifting priorities of purchasers, be it the individual, an insurance company or the state, about what care is funded.

The combination of the best available evidence and individual clinical expertise provides us with the opportunity to improve the outcome of dental health care for our patients. How good we are is no indication of how good we could be. To systematically and successfully improve our patient care, we, as members of the dental team, need to take advantage of the support that is available and consider embracing the methods of evidence based health care.

References

1. Lawrence A, Is evidence based dentistry just another piece of jargon? *Dental Profile* (2000) **29**:20–21.
2. Coiera E, The Internet's challenge to health care provision, *BMJ* (1996) **312**:3–4.
3. Evidence based website produced by Derek Richards, Director of the Centre for Evidence Based Dentistry. Institute of Health Sciences, Oxford. http://www.ihs.ox.ac.uk/cebd/
4. Cochrane Oral Health Group. http://www.cochrane-oral.man.ac.uk
5. Crombie, IK, *The Pocket Guide to Critical Appraisal* (BMJ Publishing Group: London, 1996).
6. Greenhalgh, T, *How to Read a Paper: The Basis of Evidence Based Medicine* (BMJ Publishing Group: London, 1997).
7. CASP. Critical Appraisal Skill Programme, Oxford, England.
8. Wakefield AJ, Montgomery SM, Measles, mumps, rubella vaccine: through a glass, darkly, *Adverse Drug React Toxicol Rev* (2000) **19**: 265–283.
9. Peltola H, Patja A, Leinikki P et al, No evidence for measles, mumps and rubella vaccine-associated inflammatory bowel disease or autism in a 14 year prospective study, *Lancet* (1998) **351**:1327–1328.
10. Abt E, Evidence based dentistry: an overview of a new approach to dental practice, *Gen Dent* (1999) **7**:369–373.
11. Sackett DL, Rosenberg WC, Gray JAM et al, Evidence based medicine: What it is and what it isn't, *BMJ* (1996) **312**:71–72.
12. Green SB, Byar DP, Using observational data from registries to compare treatments: the fallacy of omnimetrics, *Stat Med* (1984) **3**:361–370.
13. Harrison JE, Ashby D, Lennon MA, An analysis of papers published in the British and European journals of orthodontics, *Br J Orthod* (1996) **23**:203–209.
14. Field MJ, Lohe KN, *Guidelines to Clinical Practice* (National Academy of Science, Institute of Medicine: Washington, 1992) 34.
15. National Institute for Clinical Excellence (NICE). http://www.nice.org.uk
16. The Scottish Intercollegiate Guideline Network (SIGN). http://www.sign.ac.uk
17. Scottish Intercollegiate Guideline Network, SIGN GUIDELINE 43, Royal College of Physicians, 9 Queens Street, Edinburgh EH2 1JQ, UK.
18. Robinson PP, Smith KG, Lingual nerve damage during lower third molar removal: a comparison of two surgical methods, *Br Dent J* (1996) 180:456–461.
19. Scurria MS, Bader JD, Shugars DA, Meta-analysis of fixed partial denture survival: prosthesis and abutments, *J Pros Dent* (1998) **79**:459–464.
20. NHS North West Regional Office. http://www.193.32.28.83/nwro/pcdental.htm
21. The Department of Health. http://www.doh.gov.uk/research/index.htm
22. NHS North West Regional Office. http://www.193.32.28.83/nwro/primh.htm
23. The Faculty of General Dental Practitioners, The Royal College of Surgeons, England. http://www.rcseng.ac.uk/public/fgdp/fgdp.htm
24. The British Dental Association. http://www.bda-dentistry.org.uk/dentist/research/index.html
25. World Health Organization. http://www.who.dk/country/country.htm
26. World Health Organization. http://www.euphin.dk/hfa/Phfa.asp
27. Kay EJ, Locker D, Is dental health education effective? A systematic review of current evidence, *Community Dent Oral Epidemiol* (1996) **4**:231–235.

chapter 11

What are the implications for training and continuing professional education?

Jan Clarkson and Jim Rennie

Training and continuing professional development (CPD) for healthcare professionals are considered to be important strategic instruments for improving health.[1] Around the world, regulatory bodies in dentistry recognize that quality training and access to effective CPD contribute to improved standards of healthcare, as well as promoting the recruitment, motivation and retention of high-quality staff. At an individual level, encouragement to keep up to date with new information and modern practice comes from a number of directions, including professional colleagues, patients, dental assurance schemes, dental professional organizations, governments, and the individual's own desire not to be performing less than his/her own best. To ensure dental professionals are presented with current evidence of best practice, it is important that those involved in training can describe the evidence base and discuss how this information can, when combined with clinical expertise, improve standards of oral care. Internationally, increasing resources are being made available for training and for CPD, which, if added to the individual's investment of time, represents considerable expenditure. As with other interventions in healthcare, the effectiveness of training and CPD requires evaluation to demonstrate effective use of resources.

The concept of life-long learning and the need for continuing education are based on the recognition that dental professionals do not acquire all of the knowledge they need to support a meaningful career as an independent practitioner solely from undergraduate education. Inclusion in undergraduate training of skills such as questioning enquiry, critical appraisal, decision making, use of evidence based decision support and interpretation of evidence with consideration of a patient is not universal, but is urgently needed. Professional competence requires that clinical skills should be maintained and developed in line with the nature of the individual's clinical practice.

There is a shortage of clinicians able to deliver clinical evidence based teaching, and most are academics. In addition there is a shortage of information on using evidence in 'real' dental practice that can inform teaching. In order for evidence based healthcare to be incorporated into education and translated into practice, there are two essential prerequisites. Evidence has to be available in an accessible form and the skills required to interpret the evidence need to be learned. For undergraduate and postgraduate educators, a readily available and updated source of synthesized evidence would be a significant improvement. Currently, there are few areas of dentistry where evidence has been synthesized in a high-quality way, yet a comparatively small investment from the international community, if approached in an efficient way, could rectify this situation. However, there would still need to be a change in thinking for this evidence to be incorporated effectively into dental education. Training would be necessary for educators in all spheres of dental education. Whereas efforts could focus on equipping the educators and supporting training, alternatively, third-party funders could influence the adoption of evidence based dentistry through decisions on what and how oral healthcare is remunerated. It is therefore important that developments in education and service are evaluated to identify the most cost-effective way of improving the quality of patient care.

A recent systematic review of evidence based practice training concluded that although generally supportive of the benefits of such training, the designs of the evaluations were such that the results were likely to have been prone to substantial bias.[2] The need to develop validated tools to measure the effects of training in evidence based healthcare has been recognized, although at present no tool is specific to dentistry. Current outcome measures focus on acquired knowledge and skills to access and interpret evidence. The largest gap in evidence of the effectiveness of training is the quantification of how clinical decision making and patient outcomes are affected. A systematic review of the cost-effectiveness of CPD in medicine found only nine studies which included an economic evaluation,[3] compared to the 100 trials included in a review on other outcomes of CPD.[4,5] The nine trials varied in quality and used ambiguous economic terms; therefore, the conclusion of the review is that more cost-effectiveness studies are urgently required, with greater attention to methodology.

Within both undergraduate education and continuing professional development there are increasing numbers of courses and training opportunities for individuals to learn skills related to implementing evidence based dentistry. All educators require evidence about how best to teach these skills. A Cochrane systematic review of teaching critical appraisal skills in healthcare settings[6] concludes that the available evidence demonstrates that teaching this topic has positive effects on participants' knowledge, but the evidence supporting all outcomes is weakened by the generally poorly designed, executed and reported studies. Only one study in the review met the inclusion criteria; therefore, the validity of drawing general conclusions about the effects of teaching critical appraisal is debatable. Large gaps exist in the evidence as to whether such teaching affects decision making or patient outcomes. It is also unclear whether the size of the benefit seen is large enough to be of practical significance, or whether this varies according to participant background or teaching method. Firmly embedding critical appraisal in a wider package of skills that also includes question identification and literature retrieval is more likely to help the use of research, rather than expecting that critical appraisal alone is necessary.[7]

The introduction of mandatory re-certification for the dental profession has started in the United Kingdom and is being considered in other countries. The educationally based system being introduced by the General Dental Council (GDC) places responsibility on the individual and fits well with the United Kingdom government's requirements for clinical governance and life-long learning. Also, the main stakeholders in the United Kingdom, particularly the British Dental Association and the Royal Colleges, played an important part in helping to bring forward a system which is manageable and professionally led. The challenge of any such system is to obtain maximum benefit, for dentists, for members of the dental team and for patients. The GDC has provided a framework and has made it clear that it expects the system to evolve with time, which it must do to meet the ever-changing challenges of a primary-care-led dental service. This life-long learning has been designed to take account of the professional needs of dentists and their normal working patterns. Where dental practices already encompass appraisal of patient care and management, this can be embraced by the scheme. In other cases, dental team members are able to use professional judgement to participate in the kind of activity they believe to be the most benefi-cial. In the United States, the Commission on Dental Accreditation's accreditation programme ensures that quality education is available and provided for dentists, dental specialists, and allied dental personnel.

Many dismiss this form of system as meaningless hour counting, which will not improve dentists' knowledge or patient care. Although there may be an element of truth in this view, particularly for those who wish to pay lip service to CPD, a more considered view is to recognize that a statutory framework gives those who manage postgraduate dental education an exciting opportunity to maximize the outcomes from CPD. One obvious positive outcome would be to demonstrate that participa-tion in postgraduate education is cost effective in improving patient care. All who take part in the organization and delivery of education believe that we do benefit patient care, but demonstrating the effect of postgraduate education is not easy and has taxed many.[3,4]

Outcome of participation in postgraduate education can be measured at a number of levels. One hierarchical model is an adaptation of Kirk-patrick's triangle, which, at the lowest level, measures participation in education as an outcome (Figure 11.1). It is likely that recent CPD initiatives will have a profound effect on this measure and organizers of accredited courses are putting systems in place to ensure that this

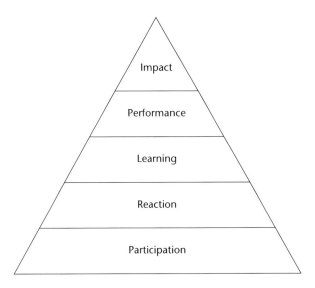

Figure 11.1 *A modified version of Kirkpatrick's hierarchy of levels of evaluation.*

outcome can be measured. All dentists will wish to show, when asked, that they have participated. Surveys consistently report that around a quarter of the profession do not attend any formal CPD events, and a variable percentage attend once or twice per annum.[8] There is a tendency for dentists to attend courses on topics they feel competent or familiar with. Although it might be argued that courses should be attended according to training or learning needs, the benefit from peer contact to reducing stress and burnout should not be dismissed.

The second level of outcome is about how participants reacted to the event. Did the dentist enjoy the event and did they feel it was worthwhile? Providers of CPD have systems in place to ensure that feedback is obtained on courses. Poor courses are dropped and poor speakers are not asked again. Dentists are busy, discerning professionals and are not slow to make their views known if they feel their time has been wasted.

Educational events should have:

- concise educational aims and objectives;
- clearly anticipated outcomes;
- quality control;

(Harden and Laidlaw).[9]

The higher levels of the triangle are increasingly difficult to measure, and there are few studies in dentistry which clearly demonstrate that participants have learned by attending and have retained that knowledge. Attempts to demonstrate this include participants completing a multiple-choice questionnaire after the event, which is marked and returned to the dentist, showing how they have performed and how they have measured up against a peer group. As a reward for taking part, the dentist may receive a number of hours of verifiable education. Recent moves to deliver education via the Internet provide another mechanism to record and measure any learning outcomes to the educational event. By contacting participants on subsequent occasions, it is possible to determine whether or not the knowledge has been retained. There is, without doubt, an awareness among educational providers that the event has to be meaningful, and that there should be a clearly stated learning outcome and that this should be measurable. This is, however, not easy, and Grant and Stanton, in a wide-ranging review of effectiveness of CPD, set out how difficult this is to measure.[10]

Does participation in CPD change (improve) clinical practice and benefit patient care? There is no robust study in dentistry that is able to give a meaningful answer to this question. There are some examples of how the system of payment can have a profound effect on the delivery of care, both good and bad, and it should be clear that in striving for the top level of outcome, education is not the only influence. In a number of studies, it has been estimated that education is responsible for around a third of changes in clinical practice, while changes in the organization, regulations and payment system are extremely powerful influences on patient care. There is little point attending educational events if the system of payment or the regulations militate against implementation. A whole-systems approach is required in consideration of this issue.

What are the outcomes of the effects of recent changes and initiatives in CPD? It seems that there is increasing attendance and that, through improved structured feedback, dentists are increasingly enjoying participation in educational events. Delivering CPD to equip all dental professionals to practise in an evidence based way requires that educators be competent in both clinical practice and the skills necessary for EBD. All major stakeholders must continue to work at those who seldom or never attend, and to improve the quality of the education, be it lecturer-based, hands-on or computer-assisted. A number of innovative attempts at supporting dentists through personal learning plans and though computer-assisted learning tools are about to report and there is little doubt that providers are pushing in the correct direction. Also, an initiative designed to promote an evaluative culture in dental primary care (by requiring participation in a randomized, controlled trial by newly qualified dentists in training) is being evaluated (ISRCT Number 99609795).

There is a dearth of well constructed studies in dentistry that examine the higher levels of Kirkpatrick's triangle and provide the robust evidence base for satisfying the ultimate goal of patient care. A trial is under way to evaluate the effect of remuneration and training in EBD in the implementation of research evidence in primary care (Chief Scientist Office, reference number OOB/3/65). Currently, dentistry goes forward by borrowing from best evidence in other fields, particularly primary care medicine. Given the current difficulty in obtaining meaningful funding for educational research generally, and the particular difficulties that dentistry as a specialty has at competing in mainstream research, this is likely to remain the case for some time. There is an urgent need for support of research in primary dental care and for the development of dental practice based research networks.

For the future, those who deliver the system should continue to keep the pinnacle of the triangle in mind and to recognize that this is a long process of continuous quality improvement. It should also be remembered that dentistry is a learned profession, and it should be self-evident that most dentists are intelligent, motivated individuals who wish to continuously improve and develop. Those who manage the system have to continue to ensure that the aims of re-certification fit with future initiatives in the healthcare systems. One way to make participation in CPD change practice is to encourage meaningful practice-based learning which is appropriate in the context of the environment of the health-care team. There should be rewards for the demonstration of good practice, and the development of effective primary care based research networks, that can be used to demonstrate the effectiveness or not of educational events would be a major step forward.

It must not be forgotten that the approach of evidence based practice can be adopted by all those involved in making healthcare decisions, which includes professionals complementary to dentistry. The issue for the profession is how, rather than whether, to teach the skills needed to practise in an evidence based way. The paucity of quality educational research reflects the lack of prestige in this field compared with bio-medical research. Findings from research are often either translated slowly into appropriate changes in practice or not at all. With the increasing emphasis on continuing professional development and the associated costs of education, to both national bodies and individuals, the gaps in evidence of effectiveness of learning could be viewed as a greater priority than some clinical topics for research.

Activities chosen as part of CPD may include independent study of literature, staff training, and background research, so there are opportunities for dental team members to spend time searching the basic literature.

A study on Continuing Professional Guideline implementation strategies and reviews of such studies, emphasizing randomized, controlled trials and trials that objectively measured physicians' performance or healthcare outcomes, found serious deficiencies in uptake. Traditional continuing medical education and mailings were found to be only poorly effective; audit and feedback, especially concurrent, targeted to specific providers and delivered by peers or opinion leaders to be moderately effective; and reminder systems, academic detailing and multiple interventions were relatively strong.[11]

Education must make dentists receptive to change and improvement and pay attention to appraisal skills: this is an area that has taken low priority in traditional courses. However, the General Dental Council's Continuing Professional Development scheme went live in January 2002, making CPD compulsory for dentists to stay registered. The organization is also working towards the introduction of 'revalidation' in the future.[12] This will mean that all dental professionals will have to demonstrate, on a regular basis, their fitness for continuing GDC registration. Best practice can also be implemented through quality assurance activities, such as clinical audit.

References

1. The Royal Colleges of Physicians, *Continuing medical education for the trained physician: recommendations for the introduction and implementation of a CME system* (The Royal Colleges of Physicians of Edinburgh, Glasgow and London, 1994).
2. Taylor R, Reeves B, Ewings P et al, Systematic review of the effectiveness of critical appraisal skills training for clinicians, *Med Educ* (2000) **34**:120–125.
3. Brown CA, Belfield CR, Field SJ, Cost effectiveness of continuing professional development in health care: a critical review of the evidence, *BMJ* (2002) **324**:652–655.
4. Davis DA, Thompson MA, Oxman AD et al, Changing physician performance: a systematic review of the effect of continuing medical education strategies, *JAMA* (1995) **274**:700–705.
5. Davis D, Does CME work? An analysis of the effect of educational activities on physician performance or health care outcomes, *Int J Psychiatry Med* (1998) **28**:21–39.
6. Parkes J, Hyde C, Deeks J et al, *Teaching critical appraisal skills in health care settings* (Update Software Ltd, The Cochrane Library, 2002, Issue 1).
7. Sackett DL, Richardson WS, Rosenberg WM et al, *Evidence-based medicine, how to practice and teach EBM* (Churchill Livingstone: Edinburgh, 1997).
8. Leggate M, Russell EM, Attitudes and trends of primary care dentists to continuing professional development, *Br Dent J* (2002) In press.
9. Harden RM, Laidlaw JM, Effective continuing education: the CRISIS criteria *Med Educ* (1992) **26**:408–422.
10. Grant J, Stanton F, *The effectiveness of continuing professional development*, The Joint Centre for Education in Medicine: London (republished ASME: Edinburgh, January 2000).
11. Davis DA, Taylor-Vaisey A, Translating guidelines into practice: a systematic review of theoretic concepts, practical experience and research evidence in the adoption of clinical practice guidelines, *CMAJ* (1997) **157**:408–416.
12. General Dental Council website http://www.gdc-uk.org/

chapter 12

Implications of evidence based health care for education, research, and dental practice

Amid I Ismail

The previous chapters have succinctly described the process of defining clinically relevant questions and conducting systematic reviews and meta-analyses. A major goal of evidence based health care (or evidence based dentistry) is the translation and dissemination of findings of systematic reviews into clinical practice, education or research. The objective of this chapter is to describe and discuss the implications of following an evidence based approach in dental education, research and clinical practice. This chapter also outlines the different approaches that can be used to translate and disseminate findings from systematic reviews.

Evidence based health care (EBHC)

Evidence based health care (EBHC) is a four-step iterative process. The first step in implementing EBHC is to define a set of clinically relevant and focused questions and find answers that may affect dental education and practice. The objective of systematic reviews is to answer questions by locating and synthesizing the 'best evidence'. Best evidence can be obtained, depending on the question and the availability of evidence, from the following: randomized, controlled clinical trials; non-randomized, controlled clinical trials; cohort studies; case–control studies; crossover studies; cross-sectional studies; case studies; or, in the absence of scientific evidence, the consensus opinion of experts in appropriate fields of research or clinical practice. The second step in the EBHC process focuses on systematically conducting searches for all studies, published or unpublished, in all languages and databases, that may help to answer a clinically relevant question. After selecting, summarizing, and synthesizing all relevant studies that directly answer a focused clinical question, the strength of the available scientific evidence is graded using predefined criteria, and qualitative or quantitative analyses are conducted. Conclusions on the quality and strength of evidence are made, and gaps in the knowledge base that require further research are identified. The third step of the EBHC process focuses on translating the findings from systematic reviews into clinical practice guidelines, standards of care and clinical protocols. This important step in practising EBHC aims to integrate the best evidence with clinical experience and the logistics of patient care. Regardless of the method used, the primary goal should be to develop a system that can assist healthcare educators and practitioners in providing the most appropriate, compassionate, and ethical care to the public. The final step of the EBHC process involves assessing the healthcare outcomes following the findings of the previously outlined steps. The EBHC process, if used as described in this book, would help educators to present the best available scientific evidence to their students and assist practitioners in making the best-informed decisions for their patients. The EBHC process represents a new paradigm for dental educators, practitioners and researchers.

Paradigms in dental education

The current paradigm
Developing and implementing evidence based curricula and policies for

clinical care requires an understanding of the current paradigms used in dental education. In the current paradigm for training dental practitioners, which was developed in the first quarter of the twentieth century,[1] dental curricula strongly emphasize the biological basis of health and disease and technical skills in clinical practice. The dental curricula can be divided into three distinct components. The first component focuses on the biological sciences that are usually taught early in the education of dental students (the first two years). The second component, also taught during the first two to three years, focuses on developing preclinical technical skills in restorative dentistry, prosthodontics, orthodontics, and paediatric dentistry. The third component focuses on developing clinical skills to diagnose and manage oral diseases and conditions. Although there has not yet been a scientific evaluation of the current dental education model, anecdotal evidence and expert opinion indicate that the link between the biological sciences and clinical education and practice is weak.[2] Translation of biological information, such as managing dental caries as an infectious disease, has been weak or non-existent in most dental schools.[2] Additionally, there are no indications that the current clinical curricula have developed scientific thinking skills among dental students. There is a definite need for a new model that translates biological knowledge into clinical practice, and develops dental professionals who understand the scientific basis for oral health care.

A new paradigm: evidence based dental education

The evidence based model of education and practice has been implemented neither in dental education nor in clinical practice. However, the potential outcomes of developing and implementing such a model should be welcomed by dental educators if they wish to move from the current focus on developing technical skills, using a regimented training model, to a more scientific and health-focused model. In the evidence based dental education model, the emphasis would be on the up-to-date scientific basis for dental care. The mission of dental curricula should be to develop dental practitioners who are well trained in understanding, evaluating, and applying scientific evidence in patient care.

Advantages and implications of evidence based dental education

In the evidence based dental education model, the scientific basis for dental curricula must be findings from systematic reviews, because these reviews, as has been described in the previous chapters, provide the least biased and most critical evaluation of all available evidence. Systematic reviews provide up-to-date information for dental educators, students, and practitioners. Systematic reviews could replace textbooks as sources for information on diagnostic tests, therapy (prevention), and prognosis. Textbooks will remain useful for describing how to perform dental procedures. Hence, a major benefit of conducting systematic reviews is the development of concise syntheses of all evidence relevant to solving clinical problems. Given the large number of new articles published in dental journals each year, it is impossible for educators, practitioners or researchers (especially in countries where access to dental journals is limited because of cost and access to libraries) to read all emerging evidence relevant to a specific area of dental care. The synthesized and updated evidence that is published in a systematic review alleviates this problem and provides a new tool to assist dental educators and practitioners around the world.

For international dental education, the EBHC model provides easier access to current reviews of clinically relevant questions via the World Wide Web (WWW). Learning in the evidence based dental education model focuses on preparing practitioners who can evaluate the quality of the scientific evidence available to answer clinical questions. In such a model, dental educators change their role from that of providers of facts to that of scholars who engage students in discussion on the content and quality of the scientific evidence. For such models to be successful, learning will take place to a lesser extent in the lecture room and more often in discussion sessions, problem-based learning seminars, and clinical case-based discussions.

Adopting an evidence based dental education model would require the re-education of dental educators and some significant organizational and cultural changes in schools or colleges of dentistry. In the evidence based dental education model, dental educators require to learn new skills to be able to critically appraise the evidence as well as the quality of published systematic reviews. More importantly, dental educators need to learn to work with clinical uncertainties, because not all questions in clinical dentistry have definite, scientifically based answers. Most importantly, dental administrators should reward faculty for practising evidence based health and they should endorse the concept of scholarship where the conveyance of knowledge is as important as, if not more so than, generating new knowledge through conducting primary research. When systematic reviews find no evidence to answer a clinically relevant question, educators must state this fact to their students and patients. The lack of evidence should provide a unique opportunity to develop consensus statements as well as research agendas to enrich the scientific basis for education and practice. In the evidence based model of dental education, the emphasis shifts from the 'message' to the scientific basis supporting or refuting the message. Dental educators who follow the evidence based model may develop students who value their scientific critical thinking skills as well as their surgical skills. Students and faculty should feel comfortable debating the scientific basis for clinical decisions.

In order to adopt an evidence based dental education model, there will need to be a change in the current organizational systems used in dental education. In the admission process, there will be a need to recruit students who are interested in critical thinking and who are comfortable with uncertainty in knowledge and seek to find answers. Skills in scientific thinking, the use of the scientific method, critical appraisal, statistics, and communication will be required to succeed in dental schools that adopt an evidence based model of education. Faculty will be required to develop skills in critical appraisal, critical thinking, and teaching methods. These skills, however, would be better gained during graduate or postgraduate training.

Scholarship is the foundation of university education. In university based dental education all educators must be scholars, but not all educators should be researchers. A dental scholar is a learned faculty member who devotes his/her time to advanced study, evaluation, and dissemination of knowledge in a specific field. Scholarship in universities during the twentieth century has focused on research or generating new knowledge. The dissemination of knowledge has received limited attention and recognition.[3] Several medical schools in the USA have proposed changing the definition of scholarship to include scholarship of discovery, scholarship of integration, scholarship of application, and the scholarship of teaching.[4-9] The methods described in this book can contribute to invigorating the careers of clinical faculty who are not interested in laboratory based research and may open an opportunity to schools of dentistry that do not have the resources to develop laboratory-focused research.

The change in scholarship and learning will definitely have an impact on dental care. In most dental schools' clinics, the focus is on teaching students to perform technical skills such as restoring teeth, extraction of teeth, fabrication of dentures, and performing non-surgical or surgical periodontal care. In an evidence based model of education, teaching technical skills is not sufficient for preparing the next generation of dentists or dental hygienists. Educating life-long learners requires training in and application of the EBHC model in dental education and practice. Achieving this goal requires rapid access to information from systematic reviews, which can be secured via the WWW, and calibration/training of part-time and full-time faculty. Such an endeavour is time consuming and costly, but, nonetheless, is urgently required in all dental schools worldwide.

The preceding discussion has focused on a number of changes to develop new types of dental educators. In my opinion, this is the major implication of an evidence based approach to dental education. Change is not easy and it requires visionary leaders. These leaders should accept and understand the need for change in the models of dental education. A major effort of promoters of the evidence based dental education model should focus on educating all decision makers, including university administrators, deans, and dental educators. The leaders in this new model should be able to develop shared visions for their institutions; develop systems for education, research, and practice that seek and welcome feedback; critical thinking; and scholarship by dental educators.

Impact of evidence based health care on research

Research is a systematic method of inquiry. The process for conducting systematic reviews follows the same steps that are followed in good research studies. Research methods are used to solve problems. The process starts with developing a hypothesis that proposes an explanation or a solution to a problem. To test their proposed hypotheses, researchers design experiments (randomized, controlled trials or controlled clinical trials); conduct surveys (cross-sectional or retrospective studies); follow cohorts of individuals over time (longitudinal or prospective studies), design case–control studies to ascertain past or current exposures to risk factors; or audit charts. Research involves more than conducting studies in laboratories. The model depicted in Figure 12.1 presents an integrated schema of how the different research

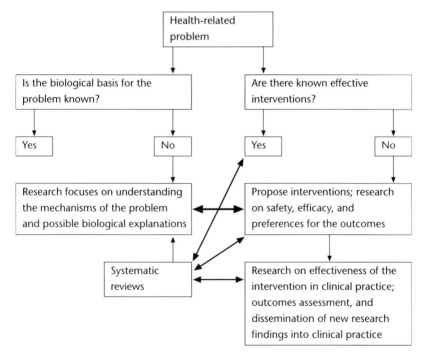

Figure 12.1 *A schema for use of research and systematic reviews in solving health-related problems.*

disciplines can investigate different issues of the same problem. A clinical problem may raise questions about the biological understanding of a disease process or the need to explain a clinical phenomenon.

Biological research can provide insights into finding new solutions to clinical problems. Hypothesized solutions should be tested in controlled clinical studies that investigate the efficacy of any proposed intervention. If a proposed intervention is efficacious, studies will be needed to test the effectiveness under real-life conditions, and to evaluate the outcomes of care (for example, the impact on quality of life and cost of care). Each of these different research questions requires to be solved using appropriate designs and measurement methods. Systematic reviews can be conducted to ascertain the status of evidence in support of an intervention. These reviews can also generate new questions for biological and clinical research. Unfortunately, the model described in Figure 12.1 has not yet been comprehensively implemented in any country. Rather, research has been focused on a few of the boxes in Figure 12.1. Consequently, dental education and clinical care do not have a solid scientific foundation for making decisions on the appropriate care that should be provided to solve real-life clinical problems, and it should not be surprising that recent systematic reviews of clinically relevant questions found that the existing evidence is either weak or lacking.[10] The dental community does not have a strong scientific base to justify many of the current methods used in the diagnosis and treatment of most oral conditions. Dental educators and practitioners often rely on anecdotal evidence, experience, and trial and error in the provision of dental care.

The previously described EBHC process can be a useful tool to identify areas for research as well as to define research agendas. Using the information provided in the previous chapters, a reviewer may reach the following answers to a clinically relevant question (Figure 12.2): no evidence to answer the question, weak inconclusive evidence, or good evidence that can be used to answer the question. Regardless of the outcomes of systematic reviews, they usually result in identifying many gaps in the knowledge base for a discipline, and the findings can be used to define research agendas and to expand the knowledge base for a

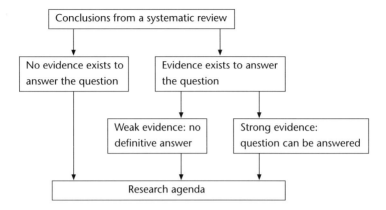

Figure 12.2 *The impact of systematic reviews on defining research agendas.*

discipline. This benefit of systematic reviews and of the process of EBHC is usually not well understood by critics.[11] The EBHC process is iterative and can lead to earlier translation of effective interventions into practice and saving on the cost of unnecessarily replicating research studies.

Impact of evidence based health care on dental practice

The goal of all health care practitioners is to provide quality care. The Health Care Financing Administration in the USA defines quality care as the provision of the right care for the right patient at the right time and achieving the desired outcomes http://32.97.224.58/faqs/mhpcompare-quality.asp.

EBHC is a tool that can assist practitioners in deciding what is the 'right care' for an individual patient. The process of provision of care remains a delicate blend of science and art. A practitioner should consider the scientific knowledge related to the diagnosis, risk assessment, decision making, prevention and treatment of a specific health condition; integrate the knowledge base with information on patients' behaviour, their preferences for different interventions, and utilities of potential outcomes; and take into account his or her own level of technical expertise.

If readers of this book were to survey the practice patterns in different regions or countries of the world, they would most definitely find a wide variation in approaches to the provision of 'quality' care. EBHC may not resolve these variations; however, the steps described in this book can help educators and practitioners to provide scientifically validated health care.

For most of the twentieth century, dental practitioners have focused on the technical aspects of care. How well does a restoration fit a cavity or a crown fit a tooth? In other words, their focus has been on the 'doing it right' part of the quality healthcare definition. However, providing a technically superior restoration for a tooth that does not need a restoration at all should be considered the lowest quality of dental care. Hence, dental practitioners need to consider other issues, such as whether the care is needed and what is the best evidence supporting each potential intervention.

Synthesizing the 'best evidence', using the methods described in this book, represents the current standard that should be followed by dental educators and practitioners. The practice of EBHC does not require that dental practitioners conduct their own systematic reviews or critical appraisals. Instead, they are expected to access, critique, and use the information that is available through the several databases that focus on tabulating the recent findings from systematic reviews, such as the Fédération Dentaire Internationale (FDI), the World Dental Federation, the Cochrane Oral Health Group in the UK, and the National Guideline Clearinghouse in the USA. Although these databases are accessible to most individuals in developed countries who have access to the WWW, others can access secondary sources, such as local professional publications that summarize findings from systematic reviews, guidelines, or standards of care. In the twenty-first century, it is expected that health care should be based on accessible scientific information, regardless of the level of development of a country. Information should be made accessible to all practitioners, regardless of their location and the wealth of the country in which they practise.

The process of translating findings from systematic reviews to dental education and practice is still in its beginning. The simplest method has been to develop clinical practice guidelines (Cpgs), which are defined as 'systematically developed statements designed to assist both practitioner and patient with decisions about appropriate health care for specific clinical circumstances'.[12] Ideally, CPGs should be based on findings from systematic reviews and be defined by a consensus panel of clinical and methodological experts. Translation of findings of systematic reviews into clinical practice can be achieved as well, by using clinical protocols that define, step-by-step, how a health condition should be diagnosed and managed.

The process of dissemination is crucial for the success of the EBHC paradigm. Current evidence from systematic reviews on dissemination suggests that there are some effective dissemination strategies, such as small-group, outreach, educational visits,[13] audits and feedback,[14] training practitioners to use clinical practice guidelines,[15] reminders[16] for specific tests or interventions, and interactive workshops.[17] Ineffective strategies for dissemination include the use of local opinion leaders,[18] printed educational materials,[19] and continuing education and didactic workshops.[17] The evidence is not sufficient to reach a definitive recommendation regarding the efficacy of targeted payments for primary-care providers to promote specific practices.[20] One approach that can be used to disseminate findings from systematic reviews into practice includes the following steps:[21]

1. Develop an institutional proposal for change that incorporates the visions and needs of all those involved in the implementation process. The proposal should:
   a. analyse the target setting and group to identify obstacles to change; and
   b. link interventions to needs, facilitators, and obstacles to change.
2. Develop and implement a step-by-step plan that should be adopted by the institution and its members.
3. Monitor progress with implementation and make changes in the plans as necessary.

4. Evaluate the outcomes and communicate the findings to all the members of the institution.

A vision for the future

EBHC is a new paradigm in dentistry. Until the mid-eighteenth century the practice of health care was based on experiential decisions that had not been critically tested, using methods that protected against the biases of the practitioners or enthusiastic promoters of a specific intervention. Science and scientific thinking are relatively new approaches to decision making in human history. Using the scientific method, the knowledge base and practice of health care have advanced farther during the twentieth century than during the previous thousands of years. EBHC represents a natural progression of scientific thinking that would have profound implications on health care.

The practice of dentistry needs to, and should, incorporate scientific scrutiny. Dental practitioners cannot remain isolated from the move towards critical appraisal of knowledge. During the information era, the dental profession should embrace the vision that dental care be based on systematic evaluation of its knowledge base. Dental practice, like all other healthcare practices, is a blend of art and science. The pendulum is shifting towards more science and less art in health care.

The major impact of the EBHC movement on dental education, practice and research would be achieved by making up-to-date scientific information on health care available worldwide to dental practitioners and educators. Information can no longer be monopolized by academic centres in developed countries. The challenge in the near future would be to spread the message and develop resources that allow all educators and practitioners to access the information. Building collaborative international networks that include dental educators and practitioners would help to speed up the process of conducing systematic reviews and dissemination. The dental community needs a major effort to document the scientific basis for oral health care and identify areas where research is needed to provide answers. Clinical experience is fraught with biases and should be replaced with scientific scrutiny by dental educators and practitioners.

References

1. Gies W, *Dental education in the United States and Canada* (The Carnegie Foundation for the Advancement of Teaching: New York, 1926) 128–131,154–158.
2. Field MJ, ed, *Dental Education at the Crossroads. Challenge and Change* (National Academy Press: Washington, 1995) 281–295.
3. Dauphinee D, Martin JB, Breaking down the walls: thoughts on the scholarship of integration, *Acad Med* (2000) **75**:881–886.
4. Barchi RL, Lowery BJ, Scholarship in the medical faculty from the university perspective: retaining academic values, *Acad Med* (2000) **75**:899–905.
5. Beattie DS, Expanding the view of scholarship: introduction, *Acad Med* (2000) **75**:871–876.
6. Fincher RM, Simpson DE, Mennin SP et al, Scholarship in teaching: an imperative for the 21st century, *Acad Med* (2000) **75**:887–894.
7. Glassick CE, Boyer's expanded definitions of scholarship, the standards for assessing scholarship, and the elusiveness of the scholarship of teaching, *Acad Med* (2000) **75**:877–880.
8. Nora LM, Pomeroy C, Curry TE Jr et al, Revising appointment, promotion, and tenure procedures to incorporate an expanded definition of scholarship: the University of Kentucky College of Medicine experience, *Acad Med* (2000) **75**:913–924.
9. Shapiro ED, Coleman DL, The scholarship of application, *Acad Med* (2000) **75**:895–898.
10. Agency for Healthcare Research and Quality, *Diagnosis and Management of Dental Caries* (AHRQ Publication No. 01-E055, February 2001), http://www.ahrq.gov/clinic/dentsumm.htm.
11. Ash MM, Paradigmatic shifts in occlusion and temporomandibular disorders, *J Oral Rehab* (2001) **28**:1–13.
12. Field M, Lohr K, eds, *Clinical Practice Guidelines: Directions for a New Paradigm*, (National Academy Press: Washington, DC, 1990).
13. Thomson O'Brien MA, Oxman AD, Davis DA et al, Educational outreach visits: effects on professional practice and health care outcomes (Cochrane Review). In: *The Cochrane Library*, Issue 2, 2001a (Update Software: Oxford, 2001).
14. Thomson O'Brien MA, Oxman AD, Davis DA et al, Audit and feedback: effects on professional practice and health care outcomes (Cochrane Review). In: *The Cochrane Library*, Issue 2, 2001b (Update Software: Oxford, 2001).
15. Thomas L, Cullum N, McColl E et al, Guidelines in professions allied to medicine (Cochrane Review). In: *The Cochrane Library*, Issue 2, 2001 (Update Software: Oxford, 2001).
16. Thomson O'Brien MA, Oxman AD, Davis DA et al, Audit and feedback versus alternative strategies: effects on professional practice and health care

outcomes (Cochrane Review). In: *The Cochrane Library*, Issue 2, 2001c (Update Software: Oxford, 2001).

17. Thomson O'Brien MA, Freemantle N, Oxman AD et al, Continuing education meetings and workshops: effects on professional practice and health care outcomes (Cochrane Review). In: *The Cochrane Library*, Issue 2, 2001d (Update Software: Oxford, 2001).

18. Thomson O'Brien MA, Oxman AD, Haynes RB et al, Local opinion leaders: effects on professional practice and health care outcomes (Cochrane Review). In: *The Cochrane Library*, Issue 2, 2001e (Update Software: Oxford, 2001).

19. Freemantle N, Harvey EL, Wolf F et al, Printed educational materials: effects on professional practice and health care outcomes (Cochrane Review). In: *The Cochrane Library*, Issue 2, 2001f (Update Software: Oxford, 2001).

20. Giuffrida A, Gosden T, Forland F et al, Target payments in primary care: effects on professional practice and health care outcomes (Cochrane Review). In: *The Cochrane Library*, Issue 2, 2001g (Update Software: Oxford, 2001).

21. Grol R, Grimshaw J, Evidence-based implementation of evidence-based medicine, *Jt Comm J Qual Improv* (1999) **25**:503–513.

chapter 13

Challenges to evidence based practice

Nigel Pitts

Introduction

The key focus of evidence based dentistry (EBD) is often misunderstood. It is **not** a subject focused just upon the electronic retrieval of (obscure) scientific papers, or solely on the minutiae of critical appraisal of published reports and reviews. It **is** focused on ensuring that the individual clinical dentist and his/her patient are equipped with unbiased, up-to-date, synthesized scientific knowledge about the best treatment alternatives to choose in order to manage a contemporary clinical problem or clinical decision.

The realization that evidence frequently takes years to influence clinical practice, or worse, might never do so, means that expectations are changing. It is no longer sufficient for a scientist to carry out a meticulous study, secure publication in a scientific journal, and hope that clinicians and others may happen upon his/her findings and might be swayed by the intellectual argument. There is now an expectation that robust new evidence should be reliably and systematically conveyed to individual clinicians, in order to contribute to the planning of individualized and appropriate care for patients. This planning of care remains a clinical judgement for the dentist; EBD merely seeks to inform that judgement, which must also take into account all circumstances and preferences specific to the individual patient concerned.

The vision for EBD is summarized in the matrix shown in Figure 13.1. That is, that EBD will become an on-going, iterative, international process, whereby appropriate and relevant examples of **primary research** are taken through an interlocking matrix of activity, during which they are **appraised critically** and synthesized in **systematic reviews**. These are then **disseminated effectively** with the aid of **researchers, industry, dental-care** and **professional organizations**, in conjunction with **undergraduate** and **postgraduate dental education** interests, to be **implemented effectively** and timeously by **clinicians**

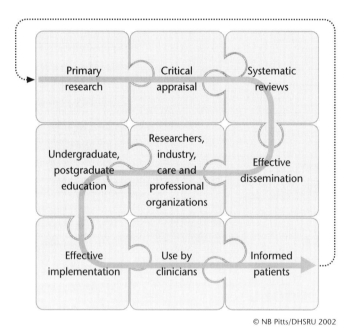

© NB Pitts/DHSRU 2002

Figure 13.1 *The evidence based dentistry (EBD) matrix shows how findings from research influence clinicians and patient care.*

The jigsaw puzzle sequence: the logical sequence that the flow of information takes is indicated by the interlocking puzzle pieces across the top, from primary research to the findings undergoing critical appraisal and being incorporated into systematic reviews. The outcomes are disseminated (back across the middle of the matrix) to research interests, care providers/funders and professional groups, as well as to education providers. From here, implementation activities are launched (across the bottom of the matrix) to reach both clinicians and patients.

seeking to improve effective and appropriate care for **informed patients**. Robust evaluation of this care will, in time, contribute to refining the agenda for **new primary research** to be conducted to a high standard, using modern and rigorous designs.

This vision has yet to be achieved. Although, in some cases, individual dentists and dental scientists have been carrying out a number of the key steps outlined above (albeit without necessarily using the more recently specified labels and jargon), there have been, and continue to be, many blind spots and delays in the knowledge-transfer process.

This chapter seeks to provide a review of the many facets of EBD, some of which have yet to be fully recognized by the protagonists, whereas others are now increasingly well understood. It will look particularly at the challenges to be met in gaining more widespread acceptance and implementation of EBD in dentistry.

The interlocking matrix of evidence based dentistry

Figure 13.2 defines the individual cells of the matrix in a little more detail, and groups the three rows into three important and distinct domains: Research and Synthesis, Communication of Research Findings, and Changing Clinical Practice.

Primary research

The outcome of individual studies, or 'primary' research, is the backbone of the whole philosophy. If there is a wealth of high-quality studies directly addressing the aspect of treatment or diagnosis relevant to the management of an individual case, then EBD can realize its real potential. However, the coverage of the area in question may be patchy, or offer little generalizable evidence directly relating to a particular clinical problem. In these cases, the acknowledgement and rational management of uncertainty, combined with good clinical judgement, are essential.

Another difficulty with existing primary research is that the coverage of clinical dentistry is very uneven. Although the Cochrane Oral Health

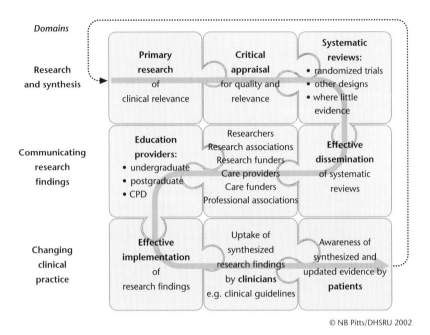

© NB Pitts/DHSRU 2002

Figure 13.2 *The detailed components that make up the evidence based dentistry (EBD) matrix.*

Group database reveals thousands of dental trials, these are grouped in specific areas and are of variable quality.[1] This patchy coverage reflects the vagaries of research funding and fashion over the past decades. Unfortunately, many of the areas of key importance to routine clinical dental practice have been relatively neglected in terms of primary research. In many countries it is hard to attract funding to support studies on such topics as, in a very competitive sphere, scarce resources are prioritized into more medically aligned, long-term or academically esoteric areas. Other difficulties encountered in redressing this balance are the length of time it takes to design, fund, undertake and publish high-quality primary research in clinical areas, and the difficulty in many countries of recruiting, training and retaining clinical academic staff to undertake such studies, either alone or preferably in partnership with primary care practitioners.

Critical appraisal

Once suitable outputs of primary research have been identified, the next stage in the EBD process is to ensure that the studies are appraised critically. This is to ensure that the findings as outlined in published work are truly valid and do not suffer from undetected biases in design, execution or reporting.

It might be assumed that all articles in scientific and professional journals would be of very high quality and free from bias. This is, regrettably, not the case, as the refereeing and editorial processes are quite variable across and within journals. However, it is also important to balance judgements about such critical reviewing carefully, to avoid excessive cynicism that may inappropriately reject valuable clinical evidence.

However well individual clinicians are trained in appraisal skills, significant difficulties remain in practising them, such as achieving prompt and convenient access to publications near to where patients are treated, coping with sifting through the huge volume of new work currently being published, and securing adequate dedicated time. There are also significant tensions in the field of critical appraisal, as expert critical methodological review of much of the existing and older published work across evidence based medicine (and EBD) shows it to fall short of modern standards of objectively measured methodological quality. It is important to establish a culture in which constructive critique of previous research is acceptable, but, equally, where useful research conducted to the standards of the day is integrated appropriately into the totality of the evidence base. Recent examples of this difficulty in EBD are seen in systematic reviews of restoration longevity,[2] water fluoridation,[3] and the diagnosis and management of dental caries.[4]

It is imperative that all clinicians are trained to adopt a constructively and professionally critical mindset in making their own assessments of published work. It should be appreciated that, looked at nationally, the size and complexity of this training task is somewhat daunting.

The critical appraisal process looks not only at the **quality** of any particular study, but also considers the **relevance** of the study to the particular clinical question being considered. Thus, a range of questions will be asked to establish whether the population under study, the setting or service environment in which it was carried out, and the particular procedure or intervention assessed, can be related to the clinical case or problem under consideration. This test of the generalizability of research findings is important in terms of the degree to which the findings should influence individual clinical practice.

Systematic reviews

Systematic reviews are the cornerstone of EBD and should consist of a thorough, unbiased, explicit, transparent and systematic process whereby **all** the evidence pertaining to specific, well defined review questions is sought and appraised, once again in terms of both quality and relevance. The care with which the review question is specified is key to the utility and quality of the subsequent review.

Until quite recently, literature reviews (secondary research) were regarded in many ways as being inferior to undertaking new (or primary) research. The balance has now changed, and it is appreciated that the value of each new study can only really be established by comparison with an unbiased and comprehensive review of the previous work in that specific area.

Having identified as much of the evidence as possible, the next step involves the systematic synthesis of findings, using robust and comparable analyses of the findings to establish the strength of evidence across a number of studies, research teams, designs or countries. Ideally, one would wish to review a number of randomized controlled trials (RCTs) and establish a 'meta-analysis', a rigorous, composite overview of the degree of success of the particular intervention in question. Given the amount of effort and time required to undertake such reviews, it is important not to duplicate effort. The international EBD/EBM community is usually extremely generous in sharing search strategies and results to minimize duplication of effort. This type of review is often led by the Cochrane Collaboration, which has a specific Oral Health Group that maintains a register of randomized trials in dentistry. The Cochrane Collaboration is an international organization that aims to help people make well informed decisions about health care by preparing, maintaining and promoting the accessibility of systematic reviews of the effects of healthcare interventions.

Systematic reviews of other types of study design are also undertaken, in the UK notably by the Centre for Reviews and Dissemination (CRD), based at the University of York. Another example of reviewing non-RCT evidence is in the field of radiographic diagnostic yield and safety, reviewed in an evidence based guideline on selection criteria in dental radiography.[5] Another increasingly difficult area, given the large gaps in the evidence covering clinical dentistry, is where reviews are clearly indicated but there is little or no high-quality scientific evidence directly applicable to the review question. Recent examples include the area of clinical examination and record keeping, where the Faculty of General Dental Practitioners (UK) sought to produce an evidence based guideline, but, owing to the lack of available evidence, had to produce a good-practice guideline instead.[6] It is not always appreciated that the outcomes of systematic reviews are inherently unpredictable, as they depend on objective analyses of studies that meet specific inclusion criteria – some of which may not be well known to researchers or policy makers in advance of the review. Equally, some popular and oft-cited studies may unexpectedly fail to pass preset thresholds of methodological quality.

Effective dissemination

There has been a widely accepted assumption that research published in a journal or presented at a learned scientific meeting would then somehow come to professional notice, gain wide acceptance and later be adopted into clinical practice by the majority. In reality, the communication of research findings was (and often still is) a haphazard, variable, unpredictable and unreliable process. Merely publishing in journals has been shown to be a largely ineffective strategy.[7] Most clinicians do not have sufficient time (or the facilities) to read a number of different journals regularly, in the hope that they may come across individual articles that might be of direct use to them.

We have a problem in that, just when the proponents of EBD wish clinicians to be accessing research findings, there is a dramatically increasing volume of variable-quality research. There is also an increasing body of knowledge, which indicates that health professionals do not regularly obtain clinically useful material from published journal articles.[7] Perhaps the research findings need to be disseminated in an active way – to be marketed to different groups in an efficient and attractive format, accessible to the practising dentist. Unfortunately, in dentistry (as in other fields), little attention has been paid to this task. The culture of the research environment has been to focus on scientific publication in peer-review journals. This having been achieved, the researcher often feels his/her task has been accomplished – others contend that the scientist then has a further responsibility to promote the communication of the findings. A further tension in many countries is that researchers can be pressured into publishing only in 'high-impact' but inaccessible journals, whereas publication in lesser journals or magazines (which might reach end-users more readily) is frowned upon. A relatively simple way of increasing access to published research findings is to provide searchable reference lists on websites[8] and to use practitioner-friendly, on-line journals.[9]

Historically, many research funders and employers have not been keen to pay for dissemination activity, even though it is likely to produce a better return on their investment. A related difficulty is that some excellent researchers are not equipped with the communication skills to disseminate the findings to clinicians, the media, or even to colleagues. In some cases, marketing organizations are better equipped to undertake such tasks. It is frequently not clear who should be responsible for dissemination – that is, the researcher, research funder, or health service/organization – and this should be agreed on a case-by-case basis.

There is a growing trend for research grants to require applicants to outline dissemination activities and to stipulate this as a condition of funding. Although effective dissemination is now an area of study in its own right, the choice of method(s) employed (for example, targeted professional journal articles, conference papers, CD-ROMs, Internet posting or inclusion in continuing professional development activities) is still a largely empirical process.

Research, industry, dental care and professional organizations

Now we reach the central square of the EBD matrix – potentially a key element, but perversely, this cell contains a number of types of organization which, to date, do not see themselves as involved with the EBD process, or who are, thus far, reluctant in some way to take an active part in the process. Hopefully, this will change as a greater understanding spreads about the value and utility of EBD to a broad number of groups, with a common ultimate focus on improving patient care.

Researchers
Researchers obviously have a key role in the EBD process, and provide the core resource. However, there is still much to be done in terms of communication to more of them to explain the full range of components that make up EBD and how they can make contributions in a variety of cells of the EBD matrix. A key and synergistic link is with dental education.

Research associations
The missions of most research associations mean that their aims are congruent with the aims of EBD. More associations are becoming aware of this and facilitating EBD activities for their members, ranging from symposia to systematic reviews. A positive example is the International Association for Dental Research, which is forming an International Collaboration for Evidence Based Dentistry (ICEBD) across all of its groups. However, some associations focus exclusively on research and its internal politics, and not on the communication and use of the research findings they produce.

Research funders

Those funding dental research are increasingly adopting EBD methodology as the foundation of their activities. Two examples are the National Institute for Dental and Cranio-Facial Research (NIDCR) in the USA and the Medical Research Council (MRC) in the UK, who both increasingly require systematic reviews prior to agreeing new funding or taking strategic decisions. As funders come under increasing pressure to be more accountable for the research dollars spent, it is helpful to demonstrate through systematic reviews that they are not duplicating others' work inadvertently, but are funding research into identified gaps in knowledge, or building explicitly on existing evidence.

Dental industry

In recent years, the international manufacturers of toothpaste have undertaken and published a wide range of high-quality, randomized, controlled trials of caries-preventive and gum-health products, and have thus made major contributions to the evidence base. The manufacturers of dental materials also have a pivotal role to play in taking forward products to improve patient care, but there are tensions where in-vivo studies may only become available once a product has been on the market for some time. There are significant opportunities here for technological progress to improve oral health and dental care, and for efficient communication of results to both dentists and patients.

Care providers and funders

The individual care provider is the important clinician at the end of the EBD process. However, the provider organization, whether this be part of a state-run health service, a health maintenance organization, or, in some countries, a dental body or business, should also have a strategic interest in EBD. Such organizations need to be able to ensure that they are delivering clinically effective care based on current evidence if they are going to be able to satisfy developing public and professional expectations and maintain activity in a competitive environment. Similarly, those who fund dental care, be they governments, insurance companies or patients, also have a developing and continuing interest in defining what constitutes the most appropriate and effective forms of dental care, and in understanding how this evolves in the light of new research findings.

Professional associations

Many professional associations seek to serve patients as well as dentists and so have a similar range of interests to those outlined above. By exercising their corporate resources and influence, these associations have a huge potential to make a positive impact on beneficial changes in clinical practice. This might be taken forward in a number of ways, ranging from, for example, support for EBD educational initiatives, to partnership with dental-care funders in professionally led strategic reform of the future shape of dental practice.

This large and heterogeneous group may not be fully aware of all the complementary aspects of EBD – in order to achieve broader participation and support, there is a need to demystify the area and reduce the reliance on specialist jargon.

Undergraduate, postgraduate and continuing dental education

There is a series of historically close links between dental education and dental research in terms of institutions, people and funding. These links must be preserved, despite the tensions in a number of countries that are eroding the number of dental teaching establishments and sub-sets of staff within them. Teachers must continue to have efficient and regularly updated links with researchers and the dissemination of research findings (both positive and negative), in order to teach effectively.

Undergraduate education must inculcate the dentists of tomorrow with a sufficient understanding of science, the management of uncertainty and the development of new knowledge, for the graduate dentist to be willing to update and change clinical procedures over his/her lifetime of practice. Critical-appraisal training and the attainment of modern information management skills should also be requirements.

Postgraduate education can then build on this foundation and hone the skills of critical appraisal, systematic literature review and evidence based clinical practice. Postgraduate study should also equip students with training that will enable them to cope with and contribute to an evolving and improving future in clinical care.

Continuing professional development provides ideal opportunities for the critical review of new knowledge. The challenge is to ensure that dentists participating in courses and related activities are **open** to new knowledge, provided that it is based on a sound foundation, and are prepared to contemplate changing clinical practice. Ideally, education providers should be actively involved in research, both to keep them up to date and to build the credibility of this involvement with students.

Effective implementation

It used to be assumed that if only the barrier of the effective dissemination of research findings to clinicians and opinion formers could be overcome, then clinical practice would inevitably change. Not surprisingly, however, it has been shown that clinicians behave in a similar way to other human beings, and that behaviour change among dentists is not a simple Pavlovian response to new information or apparent incentives. There is now a considerable evidence base from medical practice on the subject of behaviour change among clinicians.[7,10] This literature confirms that there have been significant and unpredictable delays in research being integrated into clinical practice. As a consequence, significant benefits to patients (in terms of lives saved, in many instances) have either not been achieved, or have only been apparent some 10 years or so after scientific opinion accepted that a particular intervention represented optimal care.

Reports of inappropriate care abound across different healthcare settings, countries and specialties. In the UK, the recognition of the failure to translate research findings into practice has led the government to propose the introduction of so-called clinical governance to 'assure and improve clinical standards at local level throughout the National Health

Service'.[11] In response to these concerns, a discrete focus has developed upon the **implementation** of research findings into practice. Implementation research is the scientific study of methods to promote the uptake of research findings, and hence to reduce inappropriate care. It includes the study of influences on healthcare professionals' behaviour, and interventions to enable them to use research findings more effectively. This has demonstrated that didactic lectures and journal articles, by themselves, do not change practice.

One of the most promising, but complex, areas seeking to achieve effective implementation of findings is the use of evidence based clinical guidelines. Once again, we can learn from medicine and move to ensure that we are both rigorous and transparent in the methodology used to develop guidelines and communicate research findings to clinicians effectively, in an unbiased and user-friendly way.[12] This is becoming more important as the volume of new findings deserving to be implemented into practice increases, and can be expected to increase further with the anticipated maturation of genetic-based diagnostic and therapeutic interventions. It should be appreciated, however, that not all results from implementation research in primary medical care translate directly into the different primary dental care setting. Thus, the effective delivery of EBD needs to employ evidence based strategies for the implementation of new research findings.

Use by clinicians

The end-point of EBD is the practical use of research findings by individual dentists; this is both the key part and the hardest part of the process. The classic definition of evidence based medicine is 'the conscientious, explicit and judicious use of current best evidence in making decisions about the care of individual patients'. The same concept should hold true for EBD. The success of the process depends, therefore, not on any automated remote methodology, but on the skill and judgement of the clinician in being conscientious and explicit in finding and considering relevant research findings in making clinical decisions about the management of his or her patient. The clinician must also determine how best to use the current best evidence, while recognizing that, in many fields, definitive evidence will be lacking, and that the situation will change with the anticipated publication of new findings in the months and years to come.

One of the greatest challenges for a clinician seeking to practice EBD, and for researchers seeking to implement research findings, is to determine how best to synthesize and present robust and accurate information to the clinician at or close to the chair-side or in the consultation room. There are two strands to this: first, how to sift, sort and appraise the information in an overtly unbiased way, and secondly, how to manage the information technology (IT) challenges to ensure that this material is available rapidly, reliably and affordably.

New IT initiatives are being mounted in many countries, working around rapid, linked bibliographic databases (for example, the National Electronic Library for Health in the UK) and the provision of updated material in electronic form on the WWW and on CD-ROMs.[1] In parallel, guideline development activities seek to steer a course between making available useful, reliable evidence based material, and swamping practitioners with too many guidelines to read, appraise and use. In medicine, it is likely that there will be a move to the use of international-guideline clearing houses and standardized quality-appraisal systems for guidelines. In dentistry, it is hoped that the initial moves by IADR, the Cochrane Oral Health Group, the FDI and others will lead to collaborative sharing of reviews and guidelines where this is helpful. The FDI has already established a very useful listing of dental guidelines on its website.[13]

Dental guidelines produced to date vary widely in their subject matter, scope and methodology.[13] In the UK, there have been two full SIGN (Scottish Inter-Collegiate Guideline Network) evidence based guidelines devoted to dental topics published so far.[12] They have considered targeted caries prevention for 6–16-year-olds presenting for dental care and appropriate management of third molar teeth.[14,15] In England a range of National Guidelines has been published, but these have been initially produced using a different approach, and represent a distillate of expert opinion rather than the outcome of a multi-professional group considering systematic reviews against a pre-defined methodology.[16] The Faculty of General Dental Practitioners has also produced a number of guidelines, the approach varying with the quantity and quality of evidence available, for example in the areas of dental radiography and clinical examination and record keeping.[5,6] The evidence on implementation suggests that optimal results are achieved if a guideline is developed to rigorous standards on a national basis and then adapted locally to produce a locally owned guideline.[7]

There is inevitably a broad spectrum of views among primary-care dentists about the value of clinical guidelines and the relative merits of those produced by expert groups (the so-called GOBSAT method: Good Old Boys Sat Around a Table) compared with the more systematic and transparent methods. The credibility of the EBD movement is also variable among different groups, some seeing the process as an inappropriate conspiracy against clinical freedom, whereas others see it as the salvation of future dental practice.[17,18] This divergence of views should be respected. It is encouraging to note that even those who started out as overtly hostile to the EBD process seem to see some potential value in systematic evaluation of the evidence and in embracing uncertainty.[18]

Informed patients

The end-point to the EBD process should be the involvement of patients in appropriate ways, to ensure that they can take part in a more informed dialogue about what the current best evidence suggests is appropriate care and how this may change over time. In the Internet age, patients are accessing a huge variety of resources of very variable quality and objectivity. Dentists will increasingly be required to debate this information with patients and to direct them towards unbiased and robust sources of information.

If EBD does not affect patient care then it has failed in its objective; this ultimate follow-through is a test for all EBD activities. The ways in which EBD will interact with the dentist–patient dialogue will be different in different countries. The culturally accepted types and styles of dentist–patient communication vary, as do the tensions and difficulties encountered in planning and delivering effective dental care. However, the EBD format should assist all parties in securing a more informed process of increasingly shared decision making.

To this end, a number of initiatives are under way, seeking to identify how best to involve representative patient interests in much of the EBD matrix. This matrix (see Figure 13.1) ranges from the initial decisions, prioritizing research proposals at the funding stage, to involvement in systematic reviews, dissemination, the shaping of dental services and participation in implementation activities and guideline development. These developments are challenging and important. Patient involvement should be more than a token gesture, yet it is difficult to secure effective and representative participation in some of these activities.

Linkages within the matrix

In describing the individual components in order to introduce the EBD matrix, they have been discussed as if they are discrete entities. It should be appreciated, however, that to function properly there are (and must be) a range of links between the various components, and that the process is iterative. There are a number of cycles where the end result of dentist–patient interactions feed back into new primary research, in order to inform the next generation of evidence based clinical care. These linkages are set out schematically in Figure 13.3, with text that briefly outlines some of the ways in which one can navigate around the matrix.

Delivering the vision of evidence based dentistry

This chapter sets out the challenges associated with delivering all aspects of the interlocking matrix of EBD as an integrated whole, and illustrates how EBD should have a significant and sustained impact on clinical

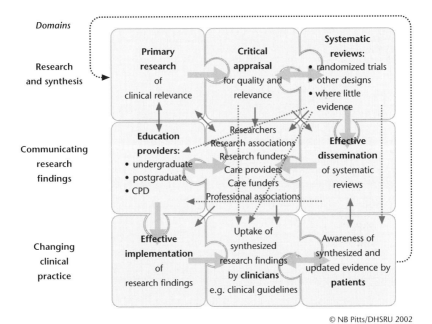

© NB Pitts/DHSRU 2002

Figure 13.3 *The interrelationships between components of the evidence based dentistry (EBD) matrix.*

Links are shown as large dotted arrows, which also demonstrate the bi-directional and close links between a) critical appraisal and systematic reviews, b) research and education interests, and c) clinicians and patients. **Other links between adjacent cells:** *It should be appreciated that direct transfer between other adjacent cells is desirable and does happen. Examples are the links between education providers and primary research, researchers and implementation, as well as dissemination of findings direct to patients.* **Cross-cell linkages** *also take place, and, in particular, a degree of direct take-up of systematic review findings by education providers, clinicians and patients is desirable in the future. The efficient transfer of research findings to affect patient care is important, but unfortunately we have yet to attain all the linkages shown in Figure 13.3 – many gaps remain. The challenge of EBD is to smooth out these pathways and facilitate the transfer and conversion of new knowledge into improved care within a realistic time-frame.*

practice. Currently not all the elements of the matrix are equally well developed or well recognized. We need to know more and to develop all of the components to an equal status and value. The number of people and organizations who have (or should have) an interest in pursuing this agenda is large, and co-ordination with collaboration will be required to reach an optimal impact on clinical practice. These collaborations must overcome the influence of the exhortations in recent years for researchers and research groups to be more competitive.

Another challenge in delivering EBD is gaining the acceptance of the extended time scales required both for generating and reporting new research and for commissioning and undertaking comprehensive systematic reviews. This is important to ensure that unrealistic expectations are not generated.

A further challenge (and a significant opportunity) in England and Wales is for those involved in exploring new 'options' for remunerating dentists to take on board the philosophies of evidence based preventive care now being debated.[19]

The focus of EBD must continue to be upon the care of patients for EBD to truly become 'the conscientious, explicit and judicious use of current best evidence in making decisions about the care of individual dental patients'.

Acknowledgements

The author gratefully acknowledges invaluable advice on the subject of evidence based health care from, and constructive discussions with, numerous colleagues, including staff at the Dental Health Services Research Unit, the Scottish Inter-Collegiate Guidelines Network, the Cochrane Oral Health Group and the Medical Research Council's Health Services Research Collaboration. The views expressed above are those of the author and not necessarily those of the Scottish Executive or the MRC HSRC.

References

1. The Cochrane Library CD ROM (Update Software Ltd: Oxford), http://www.cochranelibrary.com/.
2. *The Longevity of Dental Restorations: A Systematic Review* (NHS Centre for Reviews and Dissemination: York, 2000), http://www.york.ac.uk/inst/crd/crdrep.htm/.
3. *Systematic Review of the Efficacy and Safety of the Fluoridation of Drinking Water* (NHS Centre for Reviews and Dissemination: York, 2000) http://www.york.ac.uk/inst/crd/fluorid.htm.
4. *The Diagnosis and Management of Dental Caries Throughout Life* (National Institutes of Health Consensus Development Conference: Washington DC, 26–28 March 2001), http://odp.od.nih.gov/consensus/cons/115/115_intro.htm.
5. Pendlebury M, Pitts NB, eds, *Selection Criteria in Dental Radiography* (Faculty of General Dental Practitioners (UK): London, 1998).
6. Faculty of General Dental Practitioners (UK), *Clinical Examination and Record Keeping Good Practice Guideline – 2001* (Faculty of General Dental Practitioners (UK); London, 1998).
7. NHS Centre for Reviews and Dissemination, York, Getting evidence into practice, *Effective Health Care* (1999) **5**:1–16.
8. Dental Health Services Research Unit publications at http://www.dundee.ac.uk/dhsru/.
9. *Tuith On-line* at http://www.dundee.ac.uk/tuith/.
10. Bero L, Grilli R, Grimshaw JM et al, Closing the gap between research and practice: an overview of systematic reviews of interventions to promote implementation of research findings by healthcare professionals, *BMJ* (1998) **317**:465–468.
11. Department of Health, *The New NHS: Modern, Dependable* (Department of Health: London, 1997).
12. SIGN publication no. 50, *SIGN Guidelines: A Guideline Developer's Handbook* (Scottish Intercollegiate Guidelines Network: Edinburgh, 2001).
13. FDI listing of *Guidelines in Dentistry* at http://www.fdi.org.uk/.
14. *SIGN Guideline, Targeted Caries Prevention in 6–16 Year Olds Attending for Dental Care* (Scottish Inter-Collegiate Guideline Network: Edinburgh, December 2000).
15. *SIGN Guideline, Management of Third Molar Teeth* (Scottish Inter-Collegiate Guideline Network: Edinburgh, 2000).
16. *National Clinical Guidelines* (Faculty of Dental Surgery, Royal College of Surgeons of England: London, 1999).
17. Jokstad A, *Evidence Based Dentistry* at http://www.odont.uio.no/prosthodont/ebd/.
18. Beyers RM, Evidence-based dentistry: a general practitioner's perspective, *J Can Dent Assoc* (December 1999) **65**:620–622, http://www.cda-adc.ca/jcda/vol-65/issue-11/index.html.
19. Department of Health, *NHS Dentistry: Options for Change* (Department of Health: London, 2002). Also at www.doh.gov.uk/cdo/optionsforchange.htm.

Appendix
Using evidence in
practice: case studies

Lee Hooper, Anwar Ali Shah, Hiroshi Miyashita and Sabina Kasem

Introduction

The case studies that follow have been produced as the result of an Evidence Based Practice in Dentistry course organized and delivered by the Cochrane Oral Health Group in Manchester. They have been selected to demonstrate how evidence based methods can be applied to everyday situations found in dental practice. The process described ties in with principles covered in the preceding chapters.

Case study 1 – Lee Hooper

The use of preventive fissure sealants on children's molars

Clinical scenario

My 10-year-old son went for a check-up at his dentist last week and we were told that he has a few 'sticky patches' on his back molars. The dentist recommended fissure sealant, but, as a parent, I did wonder whether this might make the situation worse, by incubating the bugs. We went ahead with the fissure sealant, but I am still wondering whether this was the right option, and want to find out a bit more in case this occurs again.

Structured question:
Participants – children with 'sticky patches' in their secondary teeth
Intervention – fissure sealant
Comparison – no sealant (no action by dentist but observation)
Outcome – caries development, side effects

Search
I know that a systematic review of randomized, controlled trials (RCTs) would be the most useful evidence, followed by one or more RCTs, so I went straight to the Cochrane Library on the National Electronic Library for Health, using the search terms (fissure NEXT sealant*) OR PIT-AND-FISSURE-SEALANTS* (ME).

Search results
There were no completed Cochrane reviews, but a relevant protocol (Ahuvuo-Saloranta A et al, Pit and fissure sealants for preventing dental decay in the permanent teeth of children and adolescents; expected late 2002). DARE came up with two reviews, but the topics were not relevant. I will look out for the publication of the full Cochrane review, but, until then, I need some information to fill the gap. There were a good number of RCTs that might be relevant, but the recent ones appeared to assess retention of sealant, rather than caries, or were comparing two types of sealant rather than comparing sealant with no sealant. I collected a paper from 1977 that seemed to include a large number of children and that had followed up for four years.

Critical appraisal
The study randomized 84 children (aged 10–14 years) in a non-fluoridated area of rural Florida. For each child, one side of the mouth was chosen randomly to be coated with a methacrylate-type polymer, while the other side acted as the control.

Using the CASP appraisal tool for RCTs (available from http://www.phru.org.uk/~casp/), I appraised the paper:

Validity – the question was clearly focused and the split-mouth technique appeared appropriate for the study. It is not clear how the side chosen for sealant application was chosen, beyond being 'randomized'. Participants did appear to be in the right age group, but caries incidence appeared very high. Blinding did not occur for either participants or dentists (as red dye was added to the sealant). Twenty per cent of participants had been lost to follow-up by the time four years had elapsed, but this does not sound unreasonable, and, owing to the split-mouth design, both control and intervention teeth will have been lost evenly. No power calculation was reported.

Results – in the 80% of children reviewed after four years, there were caries found in 53% of control teeth and 30% of fissure-sealed teeth. Overall, 1.3 teeth were saved per child by sealant application, but no *p* values or confidence intervals were reported.

Relevance – once I have read the paper in more detail, it is not clear how relevant it is to my son, especially given that it is not known whether the sealant used is similar to the one used here, a quarter of a century later, and whether simply coating the 'sticky patches' will have a similar effect to coating all of the teeth on one side of the mouth. Also, the level of caries appears very high in the Florida population: will this increase the apparent effectiveness?

Summary and action
One elderly RCT without blinding, that may not be very relevant to my son, suggests that pit and fissure sealants are protective in preventing caries. No information was reported on side effects (though non-local side effects would be difficult to assess in a split-mouth design).

Until I read the results of the Cochrane review (now at protocol stage), my children will probably receive any further recommended pit and fissure sealants, but I will be much happier once I can implement the results of the review.

Reference

1. Going RE, Haugh LD, Grainger DA, Conti AJ, Four-year clinical evaluation of a pit and fissure sealant, *J Am Dent Assoc* (1977) **95**:972–981.

Case study 2 – Anwar Ali Shah

The case for extraction of deciduous maxillary canines in children with palatally ectopic maxillary canines

Clinical scenario

Impacted maxillary canine is a common clinical problem in dentistry, with a prevalence of approximately 2%. In about 85% of cases the canines are palatally impacted to the dental arch, and buccally in about 15% of cases.

In the past, clinicians have used different treatment modalities. One of the treatments is to extract the deciduous canine to correct palatally erupting maxillary canines in individuals aged 10–13 years, provided that normal space conditions are present. The evidence offered in support of this practice has been a paper by Ericson and Kurol,[1] referred to by many clinicians as the classic paper! This prospective study is based on case reports and led me to become interested in looking for any higher-level evidence for the problem.

Structured question:

Participants – children with palatally ectopic maxillary canines

Intervention – extraction of deciduous maxillary canines

Comparison – no extraction of maxillary deciduous canines

Outcome – improved eruption of permanent canines

Search

The following terms and keywords were used to search for evidence on the Cochrane Library and PubMed: ('Cuspid [MESH]' OR 'cuspid*' OR 'canine*') AND ('Tooth, Unerupted [MESH]' OR 'impacted' OR 'ectopic*') AND ('Tooth Extraction [MESH]' OR 'extract*' OR 'remov*').

Limits were set to All Child; 0–18 years, Human, and only papers in English.

Search results

No systematic review or clinical trial could be found on the Cochrane Library or PubMed.

We therefore looked for a lower level of evidence. Medline produced only case-report studies without any controls. Out of these case reports, the study of Ericson and Kurol was selected and critically appraised. This paper was selected because it is quoted as the best evidence by most clinicians and we wanted to know if this really was the case.

Critical appraisal

Ericson and Kurol studied 46 consecutive palatally ectopic canines in 35 individuals aged between 10 and 13 (mean age 11.4) years with no space loss. After extraction of deciduous canines, the children were assessed clinically and radiographically at 6-month intervals for up to 18 months. In 36 canines (78%), the palatal eruption changed to normal within 12 months.

At first glance the results appear very impressive, but can we really take this paper as evidence that deciduous canine extraction improves the palatal eruption of canines? The eruption of palatal canines might have occurred anyway, without deciduous canine extraction. Do we have any evidence against the last argument? The authors state that, according to their clinical experience, it is highly unlikely that this improvement would have occurred without the extraction of deciduous canines. Presumably, they had observed many clinical cases where the deciduous canines were retained. If they had seen these cases, why did they not present them as a control group? This study cannot be presented as strong clinical evidence, as has been claimed by many clinicians, in support of our clinical question.

The next step will be to carry out a systematic review on the topic, as we might have missed any clinical trials that do exist, and which might come to light through a more comprehensive search. The title has been submitted for registration with the Cochrane Oral Health Group for systematic review. However, if no clinical trial is found, the next step will be to initiate a randomized clinical trial.

Reference

1. Ericson S, Kurol J, Early treatment of palatally erupting maxillary canines by extraction of the primary canines, *Eur J Orthodont* (1998) **10**:283–295.

Case study 3 – Hiroshi Miyashita

Managing severe periodontal disease in patients displaying deep angular bony defects: periodontal surgery with or without use of Emdogain?

Clinical scenario

Mrs K (aged 31) was referred for the treatment of localized severe periodontal disease. The referring dentist has been treating her problems thoroughly (non-surgically) for years. Although her compliance and oral hygiene appeared almost perfect, there were several sites with deep periodontal pockets (~ 8 mm) and radiographs showed angular bony defects at those sites. As a specialist in periodontology, you know that you usually obtain reasonably good results from your conventional surgical technique.

However, you have been impressed by recent information reporting the successful results of Emdogain® (a gel-form enamel matrix derivative that should be applied to the cleaned root surface during periodontal surgery and which is believed to induce true periodontal regeneration) when combined with periodontal surgery for the treatment of deep periodontal defects. You wonder: 'Does Emdogain® treatment combined with periodontal surgery produce better clinical outcomes than conventional periodontal surgery alone?'

Structured question:

Participants – adult periodontal patients (aged 20 years or more)

Intervention – periodontal surgery accompanied by Emdogain®
Comparison – periodontal surgery alone
Outcome – probing pocket depth, probing attachment level, quality of life and adverse effects

Search
You searched Medline and the Cochrane Library and also hand-searched the *Journal of Clinical Periodontology* for 2002. The search terms and keywords used were: 'Periodont*' AND ('enamel NEAR matrix' OR 'enamel NEAR protein' OR 'enamel' NEXT 'matrix' NEXT 'derivative' OR 'EMDO-GAIN*' OR Emdogain*).

Search results
There were 15 articles from Medline, 15 from Cochrane and two from the hand search. After duplicates were removed, and also studies that did not compare Emdogain® and surgery with surgery alone, this resulted in eight randomized, controlled trials (Table 1).

The studies assess the effectiveness of Emdogain® on three types of defect:

- recession-type defects,
- angular bony defect treated by non-surgical means, and
- angular bony defect treated by surgical means.

Mrs K displayed the deep pockets with angular bony defects and surgery was planned, so you selected a paper published by Heijl et al[5] which related to angular bony (one- and two-wall, mainly) defects, included the most people (33), was designed as placebo-controlled, randomized trial with a split-mouth design, and had the longest follow-up (three years).

Critical appraisal
In order to critically appraise the paper, a checklist for therapy published in the user's guides to the medical literature[9] was used. This study was well randomized, allocation appeared to be well concealed, and power calculations were also performed before the study was conducted.

The follow-up rate after 36 months was 79% (three patients dropped out and the other four patients did not complete final examinations) and this may be acceptable for clinical study. I made a decision that the bias from this study seemed very limited.

The mean initial attachment level and probing depth were around 9.4 mm and 7.8 mm, respectively, and were similar in both groups. The difference of the mean probing pocket reduction between the two techniques at 36 months was 0.8 mm and it was statistically significant ($p < 0.001$). The difference of the mean gain of clinical attachment between the two techniques at 36 months was 0.5 mm. This was statistically significant ($p < 0.01$). These data were calculated among 26 out of 33 patients only, and the intention-to-treat analysis was not used. The quality of life was not measured in this study. Adverse effects occurred in four (12%) of the subjects. They are reported as 'giddiness', 'stomach disturbance', 'shooting pain', and 'gingival irritation'. They were considered to be minor problems.

Summary and points for practice/implementation

The study by Heijl et al shows good validity and the opportunity for bias seems limited.[5] This means that the results from this study can be applied in cases when periodontal surgery is considered for patients displaying deep periodontal pocket with angular bony (one- or two-wall) defects. The statistically significant reduction of probing pocket depth and clinical attachment gain were demonstrated at the site where periodontal surgery combined with Emdogain® was performed. However, these differences were small and the clinical significance dubious (measurement error inherent in the probing assessment is ±1 mm for measurements at different time points by the same assessor). This does not appear to be enough evidence to treat Mrs K with Emdogain®.

In reality, it is very difficult to draw general conclusions from one small study with only 26 participants. A systematic review of the studies that already exist may help us to understand whether Emdogain® has anything to contribute, and, if so, in which patients.

Table 1

Author	Year	Comparison control	Patients	Groups	Conceal	Random	Split-mouth	Parallel	Follow-up
Infrabony defect (surgical)									
Silvestri[1]	2000	MWF	30	3 groups	—	—	x	10 vs 10	1 year
Sculean[2]	2001	-	56	4 groups	Yes	Yes	x	14 vs 14	1 year
Froum[3]	2001	OFD	23	2 groups	—	—	x	31 vs 53	1 year
Okuda[4]	2000	OFD+p	16	2 groups	Yes	Yes	18 vs 18	x	1 year
Heijl[5]	1997	MWF+p	33	2 groups	Yes	Yes	34 vs 34	x	3 years
Infrabony defect (non-surgical)									
Wennstrom[6]	2002	SRP+p	28	2 groups	Yes	Yes	84 vs 84	x	3 weeks
Recession-type defect (surgical)									
Modica[7]	2000	CRF	12	2 groups	—	Yes	14 vs 14	x	6 months
Hagewald[8]	2002	CRF+p	37	2 groups	Yes	Yes	36 vs 36	x	1 year

— = Data not described in the abstract

References

1. Silvestri M, Ricci G, Rasperini G et al, Comparison of treatments of infra-bony defects with enamel matrix derivative, guided tissue regeneration with a non-resorbable membrane and Widman modified flap: a pilot study, *J Clin Periodontol* (2000); **27**:603–610.
2. Sculean A, Windisch P, Chiantella GC et al, Treatment of intra-bony defects with enamel matrix proteins and guided tissue regeneration: a prospective controlled clinical study, *J Clin Periodontol* (2001); **28**:397–403.
3. Froum SJ, Weinberg MA, Rosenberg E et al, A comparative study utilizing open flap debridement with and without enamel matrix derivative in the treatment of periodontal intra-bony defects: a 12-month re-entry study, *J Periodontol* (2001); **72**:25–34.
4. Okuda K, Momose M, Miyazaki A et al, Enamel matrix derivative in the treatment of human intra-bony osseous defects, *J Periodontol* (2000); **71**:1821–1828.
5. Heijl L, Heden G, Svardstrom G et al, Enamel matrix derivative (EMDOGAIN) in the treatment of intrabony periodontal defects, *J Clin Periodontol* (1997); **24**:705–714.
6. Wennstrom JL, Lindhe J, Some effects of enamel matrix proteins on wound healing in the dento-gingival region, *J Clin Periodontol* (2002); **29**:9–14.
7. Modica F, Del Pizzo M, Roccuzzo M et al, Coronally advanced flap for the treatment of buccal gingival recessions with and without enamel matrix derivative: a split-mouth study, *J Periodontol* (2000); **71**:1693–1698.
8. Hagewald S, Spahr A, Rompola E et al, Comparative study of Emdogain and coronally advanced flap technique in the treatment of human gingival recessions: a prospective controlled clinical study, *J Clin Periodontol* (2002); **29**:35–41.
9. Guyatt G, Cook D, Devereaux PD et al, Users' guides to the medical literature, *JAMA* (2002); **81**–82.

Case Study 4 – Sabina Kasem

Twin block treatment in children with prominent front teeth

Clinical scenario

Prominent upper front teeth (class II occlusion) are one of the most common problems seen by orthodontists. The aetiology is complex and usually involves a combination of anomalies in the position of the jaws, teeth and/or lips. Problems associated with these prominent teeth are the increased likelihood of trauma[1] and an appearance that patients are unhappy with.[2]

Various options are available to reduce the prominence of upper front teeth. Removable functional appliances are commonly used to treat this condition by moving upper front teeth backwards and/or modifying the growth of the jaws. Treatment is usually carried out while the patient is growing and when there are enough adult teeth present to allow the functional appliance to be worn. The aim of a functional appliance is to effectively reduce the prominence of the maxillary incisors. A twin block is a removable functional appliance, fitted to both the upper and lower jaws, widely advocated for this purpose.

Structured question:
Participants – children with prominent front teeth
Intervention – twin block treatment
Comparison – other removable functional appliances
Outcome – change in prominence of front teeth

Search strategy
Peer-group discussions were held to assess personal opinions and to identify any established papers and gather information about them.

A search was carried out on electronic databases. Terms used were: ('twin block' OR 'twin-block' OR 'functional appliances') AND 'overjet near reduct*'.

Databases used were the Cochrane Library (at current issue), Medline (1966–present) and Embase (1980–present) (databases searched to include only papers in the English language).

Search results
Systematic review – one protocol found – orthodontic treatment for prominent upper front teeth in children.[3]

Randomized clinical trial – one found – a prospective evaluation of Bass, Bionator, and twin block appliances. Part 1 – the hard tissues.[4]

Case–control study – one found – The effects of twin blocks: a prospective controlled study.[5]

Case series – one found – a comparison of twin block, Andresen and removable appliances in the treatment of class II division 1 malocclusion.[6]

Critical appraisal
A prospective evaluation of Bass, Bionator, and Twin Block appliances. Part 1 – the hard tissues.[4]

This was the only study carried out as a randomized, clinical trial.

Forty-seven adolescent patients were randomly allocated to three different functional-appliance groups and compared with an untreated control group over a nine-month period. The control group was not randomly allocated and comprised subjects that were most recently placed on the waiting list and were therefore younger, as it was not considered ethical to defer the treatment of patients who had been on the waiting list longest. All the patients were accounted for throughout the study.

Radiographic analysis using lateral cephalograms of all the subjects in the four groups was carried out before the trial and at the end of the nine-month observation period. The outcomes were assessed blind in a random sequence by two different operators. Reliability and reproducibility tests were also carried out.

Comparative analysis of the four groups was undertaken using parametric, two-way analysis of variance (ANOVA). Statistical significance was determined at the 0.05 level of confidence.

Results were presented using simple tables and could be interpreted easily. The results demonstrated that the greatest overjet reduction was in the twin block group, followed by the Bass and Bionator groups, respectively. This was also true for the anterior movement of the mandible. However, the Bass appliance produced minimal change in the position of the lower labial segment, whereas the Bionator showed the greatest amount of proclination. The twin block group showed an intermediate change.

Clinical decision
I will use twin blocks to treat prominent upper front teeth in children, as this study demonstrated that this was the most effective appliance to use. There could, however, be some proclination of the lower incisors.

Further research
The Cochrane Group is currently undertaking a systematic review. Their results may help me to evaluate the long-term benefits of various appliances used to treat children with prominent upper front teeth and the effect that proclination of the lower incisors has on the overall orthodontic management of these patients.

References

1. Nguyan QV, Bezemer PD, Habets L, Prahl-Anderson B, A systematic review of the relationship between overjet size and traumatic dental injuries, *Eur J Orthod* (1999) 21:501–515.
2. Kilpelainen PV, Phillips C, Tulloch JF, Anterior tooth position and motivation for early treatment, *Angle Orthod* (1993) 63:171–174.
3. Harrison JE, O'Brien KD, Worthington HV, Bickley SR, Scholey JM, Shaw WC, Orthodontic treatment for prominent upper front teeth in children (Protocol for a Cochrane Review). In: The Cochrane Library (2002) Issue 3 (Oxford: Update Software).
4. Illing HM, Morris DO, Lee RT, A prospective evaluation of Bass, Bionator and Twin Block appliances. Part 1 – the hard tissues, *Eur J Orthod* (1998) 20:501–516.
5. Lund DI, Sandler PJ, The effects of Twin Blocks: a prospective controlled study *Am J Orthod Dentofac Orthop* (1998) 113:104–110.
6. Trenouth MJ, A comparison of Twin Block, Andresen and removable appliances in the treatment of Class II Division malocclusion, *Functional Orthod* (1992) 9:26–31.

Glossary

Bias – a systematic error or deviation in results or inferences. In studies of the effects of health care, bias can arise from systematic differences in the groups that are compared (selection bias), the care that is provided, or exposure to other factors apart from the intervention of interest (performance bias), withdrawals or exclusions of people entered into the study (attrition bias) or how outcomes are assessed (detection bias). Bias does not necessarily carry an imputation of prejudice, such as the investigators' desires for particular results. This differs from conventional use of the word, in which bias refers to a partisan point of view.

Case–control study – a *retrospective* study which involves identifying patients who have had a particular outcome (cases), and control patients who do not have that outcome, and then establishing whether there had been a specified exposure or not.

Cochrane Collaboration – an international organization that aims to help people make well informed decisions about health care by preparing, maintaining and promoting the accessibility of systematic reviews of the effects of health-care interventions. It is a not-for-profit organization, established as a company, limited by guarantee, and registered as a charity in the UK (number 1045921).

Cohort study – a *prospective* or *longitudinal* study involving the identification of two groups (cohorts) of patients, one of which receives the exposure of interest whereas the other group does not. The two groups are compared as to the outcome being observed.

Cross-sectional survey – a study that examines the relationship between diseases (or other health-related characteristics) and other variables of interest as they exist in a defined population at one particular time. The temporal sequence of cause and effect cannot necessarily be determined in a cross-sectional study.

Confidence interval (CI) – the range within which the 'true' value – for example the size of effect of an intervention – is expected to lie, with a given degree of certainty (eg 95 or 99%). Note – confidence intervals represent the probability of random errors, but not systematic errors (bias).

Critical appraisal – the process of evaluating and interpreting evidence, giving consideration to its validity, results and relevance to clinical practice, whether that evidence comes from clinical observation, laboratory results, scientific literature, or other sources.

Evidence based practice – the conscientious use of current best evidence to aid in making decisions about the care of individual patients or the delivery of health services. Current best evidence is up-to-date information from relevant, valid research about the effects of different forms of health care.

Funnel plot – a graphical display of some measure of precision (eg sample size, standard error of the logRR, weight) against effect size, which can be used to investigate publication bias.

Heterogeneity – in systematic reviews that compare groups of studies, heterogeneity refers to the variability or differences in results between the studies. A distinction is sometimes made between 'statistical heterogeneity' (differences in the reported effects), 'methodological heterogeneity' (differences in study design) and 'clinical heterogeneity' (differences between studies in key characteristics of the participants, interventions or outcome measures). Statistical tests of heterogeneity are used to assess whether the observed variability in study results (effect sizes) is greater than that expected to occur by chance. However, these tests have low statistical power. The opposite of heterogeneity is homogeneity.

Hierarchy of evidence – the ranking of types of research (eg randomized, controlled trial, cohort study, case series, etc.) (for providing evidence) according to their robustness and ability to answer research questions. Therefore, the hierarchy will depend to some extent on the type of research question, whether it is one of therapy, diagnosis, prognosis, etc.

Meta-analysis – the process of statistical pooling of the results of multiple independent studies. Such analysis usually aims to produce a single estimate of the treatment effect.

Number needed to treat (NNT) – the number of patients who must be exposed to an intervention before the clinical outcome of interest occurs, for example the number of patients needed to treat to prevent one adverse outcome.

Observational study – where the study is non-experimental and current behaviour is simply observed without intervention.

Odds ratio (OR) – the ratio of the odds of having the target disorder in the experimental group relative to the odds in favour of having the target disorder in the control group (in cohort studies or systematic reviews) or the odds in favour of being exposed in subjects with the target disorder divided by the odds in favour of being exposed in control subjects (without the target disorder).

PICO – an acronym to help design focused questions. It stands for Patient/problem, Intervention, Comparison and Outcomes.

Random errors – errors due to the play of chance.

Randomized, controlled trial – an experiment where eligible patients are randomly allocated into groups to receive (experimental group) or not receive (control group) one or more interventions that are being compared. The groups should be identical, except for the experimental intervention to be tested. The groups are then monitored for variables or outcomes. Therefore, at the end of the study, any differences between groups should be due to the experimental intervention.

Relative risk (RR) (synonym: risk ratio) – the ratio of risk in the intervention group to the risk in the control group. The risk (proportion, probability or rate) is the ratio of people with an event in a group to the total in the group. A relative risk of one indicates no difference between comparison groups. For undesirable outcomes, an RR that is less than one indicates that the intervention was effective in reducing the risk of that outcome.

Systematic errors – see **Bias**.

Systematic review – a type of scientific study that tries to answer a specific question by finding, appraising, and summarizing all published and, if possible, unpublished work on a topic, according to predetermined criteria. Where more work is done on the topic after the review is published, then the systematic review should be updated because the results may no longer be accurate.

Validity (internal validity) – the soundness or rigour of a study – the degree to which the results of a study are likely to approximate to the 'truth'. External validity refers to the generalizability of the research – the extent to which the effects observed are applicable to the outside world.

Index

Abbreviations: EBD/EBP, evidence-based dentistry/practice.